100 Questions & Answers About Alzheimer's Disease

Marcin Sadowski, MD, PhD
Thomas M. Wisniewski, MD

JONES AND BARTLETT PUBLISHERS
Sudbury, Massachusetts
BOSTON   TORONTO   LONDON   SINGAPORE

World Headquarters Jones and Bartlett Publishers 40 Tall Pine Drive Sudbury, MA 01776 info@jbpub.com www.jbpub.com	Jones and Bartlett Publishers Canada 2406 Nikanna Road Mississauga, ON L5C 2W6 CANADA	Jones and Bartlett Publishers International Barb House, Barb Mews London W6 7PA UK

Library of Congress Cataloging-in-Publication Data

Sadowski, Marcin, MD.
   100 questions & answers about Alzheimer's disease / Marcin Sadowski, Thomas M. Wisniewski.
     p. cm.
   Includes index.
   ISBN 0-7637-3254-0 (pbk. : alk. paper)
   1. Alzheimer's disease.   2. Alzheimer's disease--Miscellanea. I. Title: One hundred
questions & answers about Alzheimer's disease.   II. Title: 100 questions and answers about
Alzheimer's disease.   III. Title: One hundred questions and answers about Alzheimer's disease.
IV. Wisniewski, Thomas M.   V. Title.
   RC523.S24 2004
   616.8'31--dc22

2004005475

ISBN: 0-7637-3254-0

The authors, editor, and publisher have made every effort to provide accurate information. However, they are not responsible for errors, omissions, or for any outcomes related to the use of the contents of this book and take no responsibility for the use of the products described. Treatments and side effects described in this book may not be applicable to all patients; likewise, some patients may require a dose or experience a side effect that is not described herein. The reader should confer with his or her own physician regarding specific treatments and side effects. Drugs and medical devices are discussed that may have limited availability controlled by the Food and Drug Administration (FDA) for use only in a research study or clinical trial. The drug information presented has been derived from reference sources, recently published data, and pharmaceutical tests. Research, clinical practice, and government regulations often change the accepted standard in this field. When consideration is being given to use of any drug in the clinical setting, the health care provider or reader is responsible for determining FDA status of the drug, reading the package insert, reviewing prescribing information for the most up-to-date recommendations on dose, precautions, and contraindications, and determining the appropriate usage for the product. This is especially important in the case of drugs that are new or seldom used. The statements of the patients quoted in this book represent their own opinions and do not necessarily reflect the views of the authors or the publisher.

Production Credits:
Acquisitions Editor: Christopher Davis
Production Editor: Elizabeth Platt
Cover Design: Philip Regan/Bret Kerr
Manufacturing Buyer: Therese Bräuer
Composition: Northeast Compositors
Printing and Binding: Malloy Lithographing
Cover Printer: Malloy Lithographing

Printed in the United States of America
08 07 06 05 04   10 9 8 7 6 5 4 3 2 1

Contents

Part 5. Searching for the Cure   183

Appendix   195

A list of Web sites, organizations, and literature to help Alzheimer's patients and their families to find additional resources on general and specific topics related to Alzheimer's disease.

Advances in understanding the causes and treatments of infectious disease, hypertension, and heart diseases, which occurred in medicine within the last 50 years, will allow more and more people to live longer and healthier. Unfortunately, increasing age is the single most important risk factor for the occurrence of sporadic Alzheimer's disease. Marcin's grandma, Helen, is now about to celebrate her eighty-fourth physically and mentally healthy birthday. The history of her family illustrates some of the revolutionary changes that occurred in contemporary medicine. She was born in 1920 as the youngest among 11 children, with her oldest brother being born in 1901. Of 11 children, only 3 survived to adulthood. Eight children succumbed to infectious diseases that, in the absence of vaccinations and antibiotics, were deadly. Two other older siblings died in their late sixties owing to the complications of hypertension. Although Grandma Helen also developed hypertension and coronary artery disease, these disorders occurred at a time when such conditions could be easily treated. By eliminating smoking, reducing weight, and controlling her blood pressure on a simple drug regimen, she continues to live a healthy and joyous life. At the age of 84, she remains mentally sharp and is actively interested in current political and cultural events. Being in her ninth decade of life does not blunt Grandma Helen's curiosity about new things, such as her recent interest in digital photography, which she has found to be superior to print photography.

Marcin's grandma is an example of a healthy octogenarian in whom minor medical issues are properly addressed and for whom a health maintenance plan is properly executed. Unfortunately, many of her relatives and peers were not as lucky as she is. Alzheimer's disease or vascular dementia cast a shadow on the golden period of their lives. Recent research lets us understand the risk factors for dementia, so preventing them may help in saving the minds of our aging beloved ones. Although a few drugs may provide a temporary improvement in memory and cognitive symptoms of Alzheimer's disease, the real drugs that will slow down or halt the advances of neurodegenerative process have not been developed yet. The authors of this book are both clinicians and scientists who provide equal shares of their time to patient care and conducting laboratory research on new treatments and diagnostic approaches. Because the development of new drugs for Alzheimer's disease is a very "hot" area and new promising discoveries are published monthly, part of this book is devoted to explaining how laboratory test tube research is translated into clinical practice. We want our readers, including caregivers of our patients, to understand this process well and realize how difficult it is to transform the greatest ideas born at the laboratory bench into clinical practice. Even the most promising drug has to be tested first for safety and efficacy before it can be introduced into clinical practice. Cutting corners may have catastrophic consequences. An important medical maxim is "Primum non noccere": First, do no harm. Conversely, we encourage our patients to participate in clinical studies because this will help to introduce new drugs into clinical practice.

This book has been written both from the point of view of physicians and scientists as well as the point of view of caregivers. Dementing diseases are unfortunately so common that many adults will be called on to serve the role of caregiver or to give support to other family members in their caregiving tasks. Many questions included in this book are exactly the questions that we have been asked by family members looking after somebody with Alzheimer's disease or other form of dementia. Writing this book was, therefore, a little bit easier because the answers we wrote were similar to the answers we gave to our relatives. Marcin dedicated this book to his grandma, Helen, but this book is also dedicated to all our relatives whose golden period of life was complicated by dementia and to caregivers who for many years tirelessly look after them.

Marcin Sadowski, MD
Thomas Wisniewski, MD

Acknowledgments

The authors acknowledge support from the National Institute of Aging and from the Alzheimer's Disease Association.

PART ONE

The Basics:

Alzheimer's Disease and Other Dementias

What is Alzheimer's disease?

Is AD hereditary?

How long can AD last? Do people die from it?

More...

1. What is Alzheimer's disease?

Alzheimer's (*alz-hī-mer's*) **disease** is a brain disease that presents a special challenge. For many people who have led fruitful and competitive lives, Alzheimer's disease (AD) is another challenge they must face at the end of their life's path; for many, this may be the greatest challenge of their lifetime. AD is also a challenge for family members, who must provide care and support for AD patients, and for any physician taking care of a patient's ailing brain. AD usually affects people older than 65 years, and the risk for this disease increases with advancing age (discussed in Questions 7, 10, and 18).

The onset of AD is very subtle, and the disease progresses slowly over years, producing a decline in many areas of the intellect. That decline is termed by physicians as **dementia**. Typically for AD, memory for recent events is the first function affected. This usually shows up as problems with remembering appointments, new names, and new routes in unfamiliar neighborhoods and in absorbing decreased amounts of information from reading a newspaper or book or from watching TV. In contrast, the mind usually preserves memory of distant events well until much later stages of the disease.

Slowly, though, other intellectual functions start to decrease. People affected by AD might experience difficulties in finding the right words at first, followed gradually by more communication problems. As the disease progresses, speech is characterized by paucity (a lesser amount) of words, and patients have increasing trouble in understanding the meaning of more complex words. Noticeable difficulties crop up in han-

Dementia

progressive reduction in multiple intellectual skills, such as memory, language, judgment, and problem solving and resulting from acquired disease of the brain (such as AD).

People affected by AD might experience difficulties in finding the right words.

The Basics

dling tasks and solving problems that once were easy. At first, this may center on problems in solving, for example, complex job-related tasks; eventually, however, it may evolve into being unable to manage a household or trouble with personal care. This in part is related to difficulties in calculation and processing of visual information. Unfortunately, AD does not leave the judgment and social spheres intact either. Patients in the early stages of AD may show some lack of restraint, lack of insight into problems, and even weakening temper control. Eventually, even though they were once very active, they withdraw from society and need more and more support from caregivers.

Mild memory decline and minor slowing of the thought processes are typically part of normal aging. Because of its almost unnoticed onset and slow progression, AD may seem like a natural, ongoing step in the aging process, so making a clear-cut distinction between normal aging and AD is sometimes difficult. You should keep in mind that dementia is not a feature of normal aging but is a disease process. All physicians involved in the care of elderly individuals wish to do whatever is humanly possible to maintain their patients' minds sharp until the end of their lives.

Keep in mind that dementia is not a feature of normal aging but is a disease process.

AD is a very common disease. Approximately 4 million Americans have AD, and this number may rise to near 14 million by year 2050 unless a cure for or prevention of it is found. In 95% of cases, AD is **sporadic**, meaning that it's not caused by a specific genetic abnormality. Scientists can't answer with any certainty the question of who will and who will not develop sporadic AD, but many risk factors were recently identified, and some of them can be changed. Currently, available

Sporadic disease

disease not caused by a specific inherited genetic defect but possibly affecting every person with greater or lesser chance.

treatment provides first of all a modest decrease of symptoms but, within a few years, therapy to slow down the progression of AD will likely be possible.

2. Is AD a new disease? Was it less common twenty years ago?

No, AD is not new. Although the first case of AD was described in 1907 by the German physician Alois Alzheimer, dementia as a clinical event has been widely described in literature before then, including references in the works of William Shakespeare. The earliest recorded cases of dementia occurred in ancient Egypt in the ninth century B.C., among the Maxims of the Ptah Holy. It is true, however, that AD is being diagnosed now in more and more people. There are several reasons for this. People are living longer and reach advanced age in better health than they did before. Thanks to advances in infectious disease control in the 1940s through the 1960s—one of two major developments in 20th century medicine—many once deadly infectious diseases (such as polio, tuberculosis, measles, and diphtheria) were either almost completely wiped out or became treatable. The 1960s, 1970s, and early 1980s ushered in the second major development: advances in the treatment of cardiovascular diseases. Nearly one-third of individuals develop elevated blood pressure in their forties and fifties, with perhaps as many suffering from elevated cholesterol. **Diabetes**, which can contribute to high blood pressure and heart disease, is also very common in older people. Such conditions have been recognized as precursors to heart failure, coronary artery disease, and stroke. New agents (drugs) have been introduced to treat both the precursor conditions and their consequences. Invasive and noninvasive meth-

Diabetes
disease associated with chronically elevated blood sugar level leading to damage of small vessels in kidneys, eyes, and brain, and causing atherosclerosis in large arteries feeding the brain and heart. It increases chances for strokes or heart attacks, respectively.

ods for the treatment of coronary artery disease have been introduced for wider use. Development of successful methods of treating these age-associated conditions significantly raised the limits of the average lifespan. People are now living longer and are healthier. Unfortunately, extending the average lifespan is associated with new challenges, among which is an increased risk for AD (discussed in Question 10).

Also in the 1970s and early 1980s, a significant change was seen in the concept of old-age dementia and AD. Previously, the medical society reserved the diagnosis of AD for a rare form of this disease affecting young people. Dementia affecting older people was thought to be a result of hardening and narrowing of the brain's blood vessels caused by cholesterol deposits (**atherosclerosis**). More extensive studies on this subject showed that in the majority of these cases, dementia in fact was caused by AD. Also, atherosclerosis itself does not cause dementia but is a reason for an increased number of strokes. Repeated strokes may also lead to a dementia called **vascular dementia** (discussed in Question 30).

3. Is AD hereditary?

John's comment:

I'm 40 years old and look after my 75 year-old father, who's in the middle stage of AD. My father's AD was diagnosed five years ago, and that recalled for me that my paternal grandmother was institutionalized at the end of her life because of dementia, although no clear diagnosis of AD was made in her case. When I go with my father during his visits to the doctor's office, I wonder what my chances for developing AD are. I wonder in particular whether the fact that AD affected both my grandma and my father

Atherosclerosis

deposits of cholesterol in walls of arteries, resulting in their hardening and narrowing; predisposed to strokes (in case of process involving brain arteries) or heart attack (when heart arteries are involved).

Vascular dementia

second most frequent type of dementia (after AD) caused either by numerous strokes or a slowly ongoing process of closing off small brain vessels.

means that I'll inevitably develop AD. I'm also inquiring from the doctors about the possibility of genetic testing.

Familial disease

disease caused by a genetic inherited defect and running in families. Familial disease may affect all members of a given family or only some, but usually more than one person is affected.

Multifactorial disease

disease with a likelihood of occurrence increased by numerous factors. Most sporadic diseases are multifactorial diseases. Severe head injuries, apoliprotein E4, and elevated cholesterol are examples of factors increasing odds for AD.

Apolipoprotein E

protein transporting cholesterol in the brain and in the blood. It exists in three forms—E2, E3, E4—in various people. These born with the E4 form are at increased risk for AD.

Gene

fragment of DNA coding specific proteins. Most human genes exist as pairs.

Questions such as this are frequently asked by caregivers who come to a medical office with AD-affected relatives. AD occurs in two major forms: late-onset sporadic and early-onset **familial**. Almost 95% of all AD cases are sporadic, with an age of onset beyond 65 years. The remaining 5% of AD cases are the early-onset familial type. The age of onset in familial AD is younger than 65 and varies from family to family. This familial form of AD can produce a very early onset of symptoms, including an appearance in people as young as their thirties and forties. The role that heredity plays in these two forms of AD is very different.

Sporadic AD is a **multifactorial disease**. That means that many both known and unknown environmental and genetic risk factors can influence the age of onset and whether you'll develop the disease at all. Having one parent or a sibling with sporadic AD increases about twofold your chances for developing the disease. Inherited factors increasing the risk of sporadic AD are largely unknown apart from one well-studied gene: the **apolipoprotein E** gene (discussed in detail in Question 34). If only one of your parents or siblings suffers from AD and their symptoms started around or after the age of 65, their AD most likely was the sporadic form, and your risk is only slightly increased.

Unlike sporadic AD, early-onset familial AD is a result of specific **gene mutations** (changes) passed from one generation to the next. All genes, apart from those found on the sex-determining chromosomes, are inherited in pairs. One gene from each pair is inherited from the mother, and the other is inherited from the father. Parents pass only one copy of each of their genes to their child. In all AD-associated gene mutations that have been identified so far, possession of one defective gene is enough to cause the disease. Therefore, if either a mother or a father suffers from early-onset AD, children have a 50% chance that the bad gene was passed on and that they will develop AD if they live long enough. Because each child inherits separately, having one or more siblings with early-onset AD does not change the chance for inheriting the bad gene from a parent: It's still 50%.

In the light of the information just presented, our answers to John's concerns were as follows:

- You're at increased risk for AD because your father had it; however, the increased risk is only slight.
- Although both your grandmother and father had AD, they developed it after the age of 65, meaning that they suffered from a sporadic form of this disease. Hence, that a single genetic defect is being passed from generation to generation in your family is very unlikely.
- Because the chance that you may suffer from a inherited form of AD is extremely unlikely, we know of no genetic test that we could recommend. For additional comments, see Question 34 regarding testing for apolipoprotein E.
- Although your risk for AD is slightly higher than that of somebody whose parents didn't have AD, your odds for sporadic AD can be further modified—either increased or decreased—depending on many factors that may affect your life (discussed in Questions 19 and 20).

4. What should I know about the brain to understand AD?

Nerve cells

cells comprising the brain and connected by long processes that make communication between them possible.

Nerve cell processes

connectors between nerve cells.

Hippocampus

part of the brain responsible for learning and making new memories. In AD, it is the earliest area to be most severely damaged, causing the obvious memory loss for which this disease is known.

Your brain is composed of **nerve cells**—the neurons—that are interconnected by a dense network of **nerve cell processes**. To put it simply, you can compare your brain to a computer consisting of many electronic chips (nerve cells) connected among themselves by long wires (nerve cell processes; Figure 1). As in a computer, so in the brain: Particular neurons are organized in a larger system responsible for highly specialized tasks. Your brain has a special memory system, called the **hippocampus**, that's responsible for learning and storing information. Your brain also has a separate language-processing system, which is responsible for understanding written and spoken words and for generating speech and writing. The visual system carries out the tasks of interpreting visual images (what you see). A separate place in your brain is responsible for calculation and mathematical operations. Neural cells

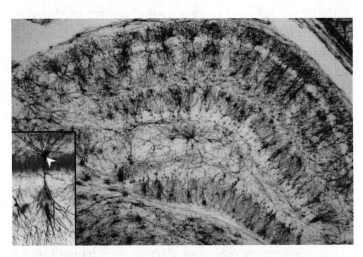

Figure 1   Magnified section of the hippocampus showing an interconnected network of neural cells. Inset: a single neural cell with a triangle-shaped body (arrow) comparable to an electronic chip.

involved in a particular brain function are located either in your **brain cortex**, which is a thin layer on the surface of the brain, or deep inside your brain, where they appear as larger structures, such as the **basal ganglia**. These large collections or groups of neural cells both on the surface or deep inside your brain are commonly called your brain's **gray matter**. That's because of its grayish color as opposed to your **white matter**, which consists of nerve cell processes (wiring of the brain) located under your brain surface. The color of white matter comes from myelin, which is the material forming the insulation of nerve cell processes.

The human brain is divided into four parts called lobes: the frontal lobe, the parietal lobe, the temporal lobe, and the occipital lobe (Figure 2). Specialized areas of the brain cortex covering particular lobes are responsible for different cognitive functions. For example, the foremost part of the frontal lobe is responsible for planning and judgment, whereas the rear frontal lobe controls voluntary movements. Language function is located in two separated areas in the frontal and in the temporal lobes. An area in the temporal lobe decodes language. It's responsible for our understanding of speech and writing. An area in the frontal lobe, conversely, encodes language, enabling us to express our thoughts by speech or writing. These two language-related areas are located on the left side of the brain in right-handed people and, rarely, on the right side of the brain in some left-handed people. Another localized brain function is found in the rear part of the parietal lobe on the left side, which controls calculation. A similar area on the right side of the brain controls the ability of spatial orientation. The

The Basics

Brain cortex
superficial layer of the brain composed of nerve cells. Most intellectual functions (e.g., language, graphic, mathematical skills, judgment) are located in specific parts of the cortex. Cortex is also a place for long-term information storage (long-term memory).

Basal ganglia
structures deep in the brain responsible for making movement smooth and precise.

Gray matter
part of the brain containing nerve cells. Brain cortex and basal ganglia are examples of gray matter. The term "gray matter" is derived from the natural color of this part of the brain.

White matter
part of the brain containing processes of nerve cells (brain wiring). It is white as opposed to gray matter, which contains actual nerve cell bodies.

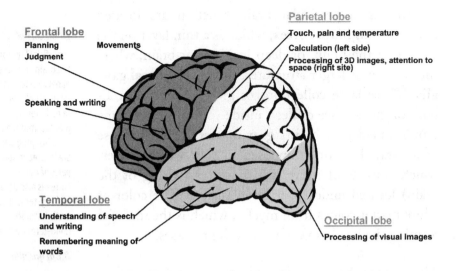

Frontal lobe
Planning   Movements
Judgment

Speaking and writing

Parietal lobe
Touch, pain and temperature
Calculation (left side)
Processing of 3D images, attention to space (right site)

Temporal lobe
Understanding of speech and writing
Remembering meaning of words

Occipital lobe
Processing of visual images

Figure 2   Localization of various functions in the human brain.

hippocampus is a structure critical for learning and making memories.

Other specialized parts of your brain are involved in abstract thinking, judgment, problem solving, making short- and long-term plans, and controlling urges and impulses. A structure called the **amygdala** is involved in your processing of emotions, linking them with images or sounds (a picture, or the voice of a mother associated with feelings of love and comfort). Still other parts of your brain are devoted to receiving smell, touch, pain, and temperature and to making voluntary movements.

With such a clearly marked and organized area of function, the appearance of a cognitive (thinking) deficit will depend on which part of the brain is

Amygdala

part of the brain associated with feeling emotions.

10

mainly affected in a disease process. In AD, the hippocampus is struck first, followed by the temporal lobes, and then the language-coding areas of the temporal and frontal lobes. Slowly, the entire brain is involved by AD, the parts most resistant to the disease being the areas of the frontal lobe controlling voluntary movements and the area of the parietal lobe receiving information about touch, pain, and temperature. Unlike AD, stroke can affect almost any part of the brain. Therefore, the cognitive deficit in vascular dementia has a more random and less predictable pattern.

AD slowly damages both nerve cells themselves and the connections between them and gradually, over a number of years, leads to loss of neural cells and loss of various intellectual (reasoning) functions. Nerve cells belonging to various brain systems show a differing susceptibility to AD. The neural cells in your hippocampus, the heart of your memory system, are the most disease-prone; therefore, memory and learning dysfunction are early—and the most characteristic—features of the AD type of dementia.

After first damaging the hippocampus and amygdala, the disease spreads to parts of the brain involved in language, calculating, judgment, and problem solving. That's when clinical symptoms from these damaged parts of the brain become evident. Neural cells that govern voluntary movements are the most resistant, so even patients with quite advanced AD are able to walk independently (discussed in Question 24).

Other dementing illnesses can damage either gray matter (nerve cells) or white matter (nerve cell connections) or both (discussed in Question 28). As mentioned, different parts of your brain show differing susceptibility to various diseases, so the pattern of symptoms is different from that observed in AD.

5. How does human memory work?

Our ability to record new information is a significant feature that allows us to adapt to new life situations. We vary widely in our ability to acquire new information; one person may record data from one category more easily than data from another. For instance, you can be pretty good with names but be poor at learning directions through an unfamiliar neighborhood. Moreover, stressful or emotional circumstances associated with an event affects the amount of information retained.

Memory is a complex process during which many types of information are being recorded and stored in our brains. We can speak of different types of memory: We have a short-term memory and a long-term memory. We use our short-term memory for ongoing brain operations, and with it we can hold a single piece of information for a very limited period (e.g., when somebody tells you a phone number and you dial it a few seconds later). For this brief moment, you store the information—a phone number—using working memory. We must also have long-term memory for learning and prolonged storage of information. Usually to remember a phone number, you have to repeat it several times. This process of learning is technically called **consolidation of memory**, and your hippocampus performs it. In this way, you can record different

Consolidation of memory

technical term describing structural changes that take place in the hippocampus during learning and allow us to learn and remember.

types of data: numbers, names, meaning of words, facts, faces, pictures, topographical organization (say, surface features on a map), and others. You absorb a great deal of information without making any great effort (e.g., by watching television or reading a newspaper). All these data are then stored in the brain cortex outside the hippocampus. In AD, early damage to the hippocampus produces an evident disability in learning new information. Because the cortex remains relatively spared until later stages of disease, you can remember old data that you picked up before the disease started and that were stored outside your hippocampus. A vital part of the memory consolidation process is your ability and willingness to focus your attention. Although the final result of a memory test (the amount of information recorded) for an AD patient and for a depressed patient may be the same, the difference between these two types of patients is that the AD patient is better on immediate recall of information, whereas the depressed patient does not put significant effort into recording the information.

In AD, early damage to the hippocampus produces an evident disability in learning new information.

Besides learning new facts, pictures, and data, we learn associations between emotions and a given fact, picture, or sound. The voice or picture of a mother or a newborn baby can bring you warm and lovely feelings, whereas a picture of a snake can result in your feeling fear. This form of learning is associated with your amygdala. Learning of manual skills, such as pedaling a bicycle, does not involve your hippocampus. Patients in whom the hippocampus has been destroyed because of a disease process may learn new manual skills but would never have a memory of the actual act of learning.

6. How long can AD last? Do people die from it?

Peter's comment:

Two years ago, I received a diagnosis of mild cognitive impairment that now has progressed to the initial stage of AD. I realize the nature of my disease and the fact that it will progress. Now I'm wondering whether AD is fatal and will cause me to die.

AD progression from the time of diagnosis until death usually takes 10 to 12 years. This depends on how fast AD progresses from stage to stage and how long patients can survive in the final stage. The course of AD, like that many other diseases, may be speeded up or slowed down. In AD patients who are victims of other diseases—stroke, infection, injuries, limb fractures—or have prolonged extensive surgery, the disease may progress faster. The same is true for patients who have limited or poor nursing care and are losing their skills much faster. Then again, good nursing care and support may delay progression of AD from one stage into another. If excellent nursing care is provided, patients may live in the end stage of AD for years. Treatment with **cholinesterase inhibitors** (discussed in Questions 52–55) also has shown an ability to reduce the rate of AD progression significantly. In addition, continued active thinking exercises may slow the progress of AD by promoting the making of new connections among nerve cells (as discussed in Questions 15 and 48). That can help the brain to ward off the loss of connections produced by AD-related damage.

Cholinesterase inhibitors

class of medications used to improve symptoms and slow progression of AD dementia by increasing the amount of acetylcholine in the brain. Their use is currently a standard of care for AD patients.

AD does not cause death by itself. Parts of the brain responsible for controlling the body's vital functions—temperature, circulation, and breathing—remain unaffected by the disease. If caregivers provide them with intensive nursing care, AD patients may live for very prolonged periods in the final stages of their AD. You have to remember, however, that those who are handicapped by AD are much more prone to accidents, burns, falls, and fractures. Recovery from such accidents is typically prolonged and not always successful in AD victims. Patients who are in the end stage of AD and are not able to move around frequently develop pressure sores that are sources of infection.

Advanced AD is also associated with restricted thirst and appetite, so **dehydration** and starvation are not unusual. This happens in part because of problems with swallowing observed in later stages. Patients with swallowing problems, especially these remaining in bed, are prone to develop **aspiration pneumonia**. Pneumonia in advanced AD is associated with a high death rate. Although AD itself is not fatal, an obvious result is that demented patients have a higher rate of fatal accidents and complications. Statistics have shown that patients with AD have a lifespan much shorter than that of healthy people. At age 65, the life expectancy is 16.3 for males and 19.2 years for females; see *http://www.cdc.gov/nchs/fastats/lifexpec.html.* Those who receive a diagnosis of AD at the age of 65 may be expected to live until roughly the age of 74 (approximately 7–9 years less than a person not affected with AD, on average).

Dehydration

medical term describing condition in which a patient's system is deficient in water. Patients reaching the severe stage of this condition may be unable to maintain adequate blood pressure and have decreased production of urine, and some AD patients may even experience worsening of dementia.

Aspiration pneumonia

form of pneumonia caused by aspiration of food into the lungs. It may occur in persons who have difficulties with swallowing.

7. How does normal brain aging differ from AD?

During normal and healthy aging, the peak performance of all your bodily systems (including your **cardiovascular system**, your musculoskeletal system, and your brain) slowly decreases. If the performance of a healthy 70-year-old is compared to that of a 30-year-old, it appears that age-related differences do not exceed perhaps 10 to 20%, with brain function being affected the least. Properly trained healthy people in their sixties and seventies are capable of performing almost as well as 30- to 40-year-olds. Colonel John Glenn, who became the first U.S. astronaut to orbit the earth in 1962, went on his second space voyage aboard the space shuttle *Discovery* in 1998 at the age of 77.

In the not-very-distant past, people believed that age-related memory loss and intellectual decline were normal developments associated with aging. Now experts acknowledge that memory loss is a symptom of serious illness. A slight decline in your memory performance and slowing of your thought process can be accepted as a part of the normal aging process; however, it's easily distinguished from AD through psychological testing that measures performance of various types of memory and compares it with standards considered normal for your age.

On the basis of many years of experience, clinical psychologists created special scales that show a range of normal performance in different age groups. Although a small decline can be seen during aging, the scores of somebody with real AD are significantly outside those in the normal range. Also, some people show no meas-

Cardiovascular system

heart and blood vessels.

urable memory decline with advancing age. Scientists are working to explain the basis of minor age-related memory losses and to explain the fact that some people are aging without any significant memory abnormalities.

Previously, many also accepted the false idea that the number of nerve cells in your brain declines with advancing age. Recent studies using more detailed methods of neural cell counting provide conflicting results. Now widely accepted is that the number of nerve cells in your brain may decrease only marginally with age but is significantly reduced in many dementing illnesses, such as AD (Figure 3). In a healthy, aging person, neuronal drop-out should not be greater that 10% and may be associated with the presence of a few AD-type lesions, such as amyloid-β plaques and neurofibrillary tangles. In contrast, people with AD show

Course of aging, mild cognitive impairment (MCI) and Alzheimer's disease (AD).

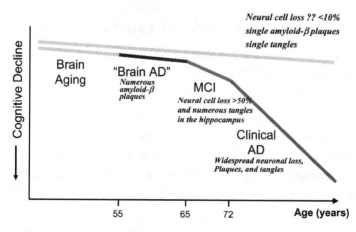

Figure 3　Schematic depiction of the difference between normal aging and Alzheimer's disease.

profound loss of nerve cells and build up a great number of amyloid-β plaques and neurofibrillary tangles. This process begins long before the first symptoms of memory dysfunction are noticed. The exact length of this period—in which the brain is already affected but memory damage isn't yet obvious—is unknown, but it corresponds to many years (the dark segment). This period is very critical because the formation of AD pathology can be hastened by diabetes, elevated cholesterol, or elevated blood pressure. After a number of years in which the disease is clinically silent, the first problems with memory start to become evident. This very early stage of AD is called *mild cognitive impairment* (MCI). Patients with diagnosed MCI experience drop-out of neural cells in certain areas of the hippocampus. The drop-out can be as high as 50%, and numerous neurofibrillary tangles are formed. The MCI stage takes on average 7 years (from age 65 to 72 in this example) and may evolve into AD, with rapidly progressing cognitive (intellectual) decline and widespread death of neural cells throughout the brain.

8. Is dementia always caused by AD?

No, dementia is a broader term than AD (discussed in Questions 28–31). Dementia is a clinical term describing gradual loss of mental functions in many areas: memory, language, judgment, and calculating and mathematics skills; such visual and spatial skills as your ability to draw three-dimensional objects; **abstract thinking** (that is, thinking about ideas); and your ability to control your urges and drives.

Abstract thinking
thinking about imaginary ideas and the symbolic meaning of things.

Many diseases may lead to dementia (discussed further in Question 28). Some of them are reversible when they're appropriately diagnosed and treated (discussed in Question 29). Examples of treatable forms of dementia include dementias due to depression, certain infections, brain tumors, abnormalities in the levels of some hormones, and vitamin deficiencies. However, a number of illnesses that cause damage to your nerve cells (**neurodegenerative diseases**) can cause dementia, and they're currently beyond the reach of therapy. AD belongs to this group.

AD is by far the most common nerve-damaging disease causing dementia. It's responsible for 60 to 70% of all cases of dementia. The second most common cause of dementia is vascular dementia (discussed in Question 30), which results from a disturbed blood flow to your brain. These different diseases leading to dementia are distinct in terms of typical age at onset, the speed of their progression, and the pattern of involvement of particular areas of your brain. For example (as mentioned in Question 1), AD has a very subtle onset, it progresses slowly, and typically it first affects memory, then language command, and then problem-solving skills and judgment. In contrast, some forms of vascular dementia may have an abrupt onset with rapid progression and may randomly damage different areas of the intellect. Because dementing illnesses are so complicated, a potential patient should be evaluated by an experienced neurologist or geriatrician.

Neurodegenerative disease

nerve cell–damaging disease associated with deposits of toxic proteins inside and outside nerve cells, leading to their death and dementia.

The Basics

PART TWO

Risk Factors, Symptoms, and Diagnosis

What causes AD?

What are the first symptoms of AD?

How reliable is a diagnosis of AD?

More ...

RISK FACTORS

9. What causes AD?

Amyloid-β

abnormal protein derived from a larger protein (the amyloid precursor protein) that is deposited in the brain in AD.

Tau protein

abnormal protein that in AD piles up inside nerve cells, forming neurofibrillary tangles that directly lead to death of nerve cells.

Amyloid plaques

deposits of amyloid-β protein in the brain.

AD is a neurodegenerative (nerve-damaging) disease. In such damaging diseases, abnormal proteins collect inside or outside the nerve cells, interrupt the network of interneuronal connections, and eventually destroy particular neurons. AD is known by the gathering of two different proteins, one outside the neurons and another inside the neurons. The protein that gathers outside the neurons in AD is called **amyloid-β** (*am-i-loyd be-ta*), whereas the protein that piles up inside neurons is called the **tau protein** (Figure 4). Amyloid-β collects in the form of larger clusters called **amyloid plaques**, which are highly toxic to neural cells and physically interrupt their connections. In AD, the tau protein is present in abnormally high amounts inside neurons, where it groups into larger structures called **neurofibrillary** (*nur-*

Formation of neurofibrillary tangles

    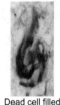

Healthy neural cell ————————————————→ Dead cell filled
                                                     with tangles

Formation of amyloid-β plaques

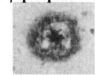

Diffuse, primitive plaque   Classical, fibrillar plaque

Figure 4   Development of amyloid-β plaques (deposits) and neurofibrillary tangles which in AD damage and destroy nerve cells causing symptoms of dementia.

ō-fĭ-bri-lair-ee) **tangles**. Neurofibrillary tangles build up slowly within a nerve cell over years until the entire nerve cell is filled with them and dies.

Neither neurofibrillary tangles nor amyloid plaques are specific lesions found only in AD; however, the presence of both of these lesions in large numbers signals the presence of AD. The current thought is that the primary event in AD is an imbalance in amyloid-β metabolism. Amyloid-β is secreted by neural cells and many other cells in your body but, for unknown reasons, amyloid-β deposits are formed only in the brain. In normal subjects, an excess of amyloid-β is removed from the brain to the bloodstream, and amyloid-β secreted to the bloodstream has a limited entry into the brain. This occurs thanks to the **blood-brain barrier**, a cell layer that surrounds blood vessels in the brain and regulates what enters the brain.

An age-related increased production of amyloid-β, its restricted removal from the brain, and increased entry from your bloodstream lead to its buildup in your brain and to deposits in the form of plaques. The buildup of amyloid-β is also thought to permit neurofibrillary tangles to form inside neurons.

When patients come to a doctor complaining about memory problems and word-finding difficulties, they already have a significant decrease in the number of their neural cells. It takes probably 10 years or more for this to occur, starting from the collection of increased amounts of amyloid-β in the brain, continuing through the formation of amyloid-β plaques and the resulting development of neurofibrillary tangles, and ending in the final death of neural cells. Researchers

Neurofibrillary tangles

abnormal structures formed inside nerve cells in AD. Their presence cause dysfunction of nerve cells and eventually kills them.

Blood-brain barrier

tight layer surrounding blood vessels running through the brain. The blood-brain barrier prevents certain toxins from getting into the brain from the bloodstream. Conversely, such toxic substances as amyloid-β are actively removed from the brain by active transport through the blood-brain barrier.

*Researchers
believe that
the AD process
may be ongo-
ing for many
years in the
brain before
the clinical
symptoms of
the disease
show up.*

believe that the AD process may be ongoing for many years in the brain before the clinical symptoms of the disease show up. Because of this lengthy preclinical course, scientists are trying to find ways to diagnose the disease in people at risk of developing AD. They've already identified a number of risk factors that may increase the chance for AD to occur. Eliminating these risk factors is one of the tasks for proper health care maintenance in middle-aged people, to reduce the chances of dementia in their later years.

10. Does the risk of AD increase with age?

Yes. Age is the most important risk factor for sporadic AD (Figure 5). The chance of AD rises sharply after the age of 65 and continues to rise with advancing age.

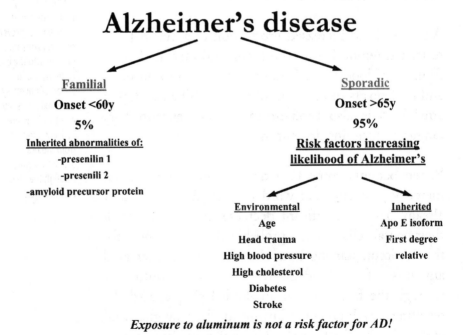

Figure 5   Risk factors for Alzheimer's disease.

Perhaps 3% of people between the ages of 65 and 74 have clinical symptoms of AD. The frequency of the disease rises sharply to almost 20% in people aged 75 to 84 and to almost 50% in those older than 85. AD seems to affect both men and women with just about the same frequency. However, in older groups of our society, women outnumber men (men on average have a lifespan shorter than that of women), so AD affects a greater number of women.

11. What is early-onset familial AD?

Early-onset familial AD is a rare form of AD. It's related to specific gene mutations (changes) and results in the appearance of disease symptoms before the age of 65. Usually, more than one member of a family would be affected. Although this form is rare, it is also very well studied. We've all heard about cases of middle-aged people who have fallen sick with AD at the top of their career (e.g., Rita Hayworth).

Scientists have identified three proteins that can have mutations producing familial AD. Mutations in these three genes combined account for approximately one-half of all early-onset AD cases (or 2.5% of all AD cases, as a total of 5% of AD takes the early-onset familial form). The genes involved in the remaining 50% of early-onset AD remain to be identified. The three proteins so far identified, listed in order of decreasing frequency, are **presenilin 1** (PS1), **amyloid precursor protein** (APP), and **presenilin 2** (PS2).

The mutations that are found in all three of these proteins and are associated with early-onset AD lead to increased production of amyloid-b in the brain. Amyloid-b is a protein that plays a very important role in

Presenilin 1 (PS1) and Presenilin 2 (PS2)

proteins associated with function of γ-secretase (amyloid–releasing enzyme). Their inherited defects (mutations) are responsible for the majority of familial cases of AD.

Amyloid precursor protein

a large protein that includes amyloid-β. In healthy people, excess of amyloid precursor protein is destroyed so that it does not cause increased amyloid-β.

the development of AD symptoms. Mutations in pre-senilin 1 are associated with the earliest onset of the disease (ranging from the early twenties to early fifties). Members of families whose AD is due to the amyloid precursor protein mutation start having symptoms of AD in their forties and fifties. Mutations of the tau protein involved in the formation of neurofibrillary tangles do not cause AD.

As has been described, if your family had such a mutation identified, you'd have a 50% chance of developing AD. Very rarely, the mutation may appear spontaneously without evidence in preceding generations. In such cases, it can be passed on to new generations. Available genetic testing allows identifying these mutations in people from affected families. These tests can answer the question of whether a person in a family with early-onset AD will develop the disease.

12. Can strokes or head injury cause AD?

Sally's comment:

My husband John is a U.S. military veteran and, as a result of an acute stroke, was admitted to the VA facility, where we're consulting neurologists. He recovered completely from weakness caused by the stroke, and now I go with him to the outpatients' clinic. I told the doctor that I have to admit that before the stroke occurred, John was somewhat forgetful and yet, though sometimes I had to repeat things to him more than once, he still was capable of functioning pretty well. Although the stroke happened to him three months ago and he seemed to recover completely from the weakness a long time ago, now he's more forgetful, and it's frequently very difficult to make him do things. Before the stroke, he could shop for groceries independently and take care of some of our household matters, but now he can't do this any longer. I also noticed that his speech is somewhat limited. He's quieter, speaks slower, makes shorter sentences, and uses a limited range of words. Sometimes it seems that he doesn't understand the meaning of some less common words. Also, when I ask him to help me in house chores, he's less helpful than he used to be. He seems to be more disorganized and spends more time on purposeless activities.

Scenarios such as this are frequently encountered in our daily practice: People will have mild memory loss and be capable of functioning very well until they have a stroke. When such patients leave the hospital, it becomes clear to their families that their **cognition** is not as good as it used to be before the stroke and that they can't any longer live independently. Similar scenarios may happen after extensive, prolonged surgery, especially after cardiac (heart) surgery, which uses **cardiopulmonary bypass machines**. As mentioned, AD can develop in the brain for a number of years before it produces symptoms that can be detected by a doctor. If people with the beginning symptoms of AD have a stroke or undergo prolonged cardiac surgery (during which multiple small strokes are a frequent side effect), they may experience acute worsening of dementia. At that point, the AD-associated neuronal loss that their brain was previously able to manage becomes very noticeable as a result of the additional damage.

The simple answer to the question asked is that strokes do not cause AD. However, the added and possibly combined effect of strokes and AD may produce serious dementia and hasten the progression of AD. Therefore, part of the professional medical care of

Cognition

unique ability of the human brain allowing us to explore the world.

Cardiopulmonary bypass machine

device designed to temporarily replace function of the heart (pumping of the blood) and the lungs (oxygenation of the blood); used during complicated heart surgeries (when the heart has to be stopped).

patients with AD is identifying stroke risk factors early and preventing stroke events.

An established relationship exists between head injury and AD. AD occurs more often among people who have had serious head injury, especially if they lost consciousness at the time. A clinical study performed on U.S. Army veterans with a documented history of major head injury during combat showed a tie between head injury and the risk for the development of AD. Professional boxers are another group at risk of serious multiple head injuries. Not surprisingly, the rate of dementia, especially of the AD type, is very high among retired professional boxers. The fact that somebody had a major head injury does not automatically sentence them to developing AD. Although a major head injury is one of the factors increasing chances for sporadic AD to occur, many people who have had a head injury will not develop AD.

The ways in which remote head injury would increase chances for developing AD many years later are not clear. This question is being investigated by scientists using AD transgenic mice. These mice are an animal model of the human AD process and are produced by genetically altering them, forcing them to express a human gene with a mutation related to early-onset familial AD. These studies have shown that a major head injury in these transgenic animals results in a temporary rise in the amount of amyloid-β in the brain. Because AD is a slowly developing disease in which a key symptom is depositing of amyloid-β in the brain, researchers have theorized that amyloid-β, which is produced as a result of the injury, can "seed" the development of plaques.

13. Does aluminum cause AD?

Norma's comment:

I take care of my father with advanced AD. For a number of years, my father was an aluminum industry worker. He retired at the age of 65, and his AD was diagnosed at the age of 72. In the past, I heard a strong notion that aluminum may cause AD. My father worked in an aluminum plant for about 30 years. He directly supervised a process of obtaining aluminum from aluminum ore and for many years was exposed to fumes and dust containing aluminum. I wonder whether his occupational exposure could have caused his AD.

No, there is no proven association between AD and high aluminum exposure. This hypothesis was put forward in the 1960s and 1970s when it was found that if laboratory animals, such as rabbits, received injections of aluminum into their brains, they developed lesions that had some resemblance to neurofibrillary tangles (discussed in Question 9). This observation was linked to the increased use of aluminum in the food industry and households in the fifties and sixties and the increasing frequency with which the diagnosis of AD was made during this period. More detailed studies disproved this connection. Closer observations demonstrated that the lesions developed by animals injected with aluminum were distinct from neurofibrillary tangles. Furthermore, researchers observed that some patients receiving chronic dialysis for renal failure developed very high levels of aluminum in their blood and brains. This could be associated with a "dialysis dementia," but the clinical symptoms and the brain lesions found in this disease are completely different from those seen in AD. Tests also have shown that injections of aluminum into animals do not induce formation of amyloid-β plaques, which are a hallmark of AD.

Most studies performed on workers who retired from aluminum factories after having been exposed for many years to elevated level of aluminum (breathing aluminum dusts or fumes) did not show that this group is at increased risk for AD. Also, most studies of people living in areas with a higher content of aluminum in their drinking water (aluminum is often used as part of the process to purify drinking water) have not shown an increased risk of AD. However, a recent study showed that high levels of aluminum in the diet of transgenic mice (see Question 12), used as a model of AD, increased the amount of amyloid deposits in their brains. Taking all data together, there is no established connection between AD and high aluminum exposure, but studies are continuing in this area.

14. Can aspartame cause memory loss?

The relationship between the use of **aspartame** (aspartic acid) and an increased risk for certain diseases was discussed recently. Some have suggested that, besides being linked to AD and memory loss, the use of aspartame may increase your risk for **Parkinson's disease** (discussed in Question 28) and brain tumors. Aspartame is an **amino acid** that is a natural element found in many food products and is a building block of all the proteins in your body. The U.S. Food and Drug Administration (FDA) approved aspartame in 1996 for use in all foods and beverages. Aspartame is an ingredient used to produce two artificial sweeteners: Nutrasweet and Equal, both widely used by diabetics and by people try-

Aspartame

an amino acid that is a natural element found in many food products. Because it tastes sweet but has no calories, it is often used as a sugar substitute.

Parkinson's disease

neurodegenerative disease striking mainly the motor system and leading to appearance of disabling tremor, stiffness, and difficulties in walking.

Amino acid

a single chemical compound used by nature to build proteins.

ing to limit their calorie intake. Manufacturers produce both Nutrasweet and Equal by joining two amino acids—aspartame (aspartic acid) and **phenylalanine**.

Phenylalanine
amino acid that is a natural element found in many food products. Because it tastes sweet but has no calories, it is often used as a sugar substitute.

As for many substances approved for human use, the FDA has performed extensive studies regarding the possible poisonous effect of aspartame. Many independent academic and private institutions also have copied and completed such studies. Thus far, they have found no relationship between using aspartame and an increased risk for AD or other diseases. Further, researchers performed studies on humans and animals to investigate whether aspartame may produce memory and other forms of reasoning loss, even if it doesn't increase your chance of developing AD. These studies also did not provide any scientific evidence that found aspartame to be harmful.

15. Does education have an impact on AD?

Studies have shown a higher incidence of AD among people with a lower level of education as compared to those who completed more school years. Therefore, such studies consider education to be associated with a reduced risk for developing AD. How a higher level of education decreases the risk for AD has not been completely explained, but studies suggest that persons with more years of schooling and a higher level of cognitive (intellectual) function throughout adulthood would need to have more pathology—a greater number of amyloid-β plaques and neurofibrillary tangles—before they developed a mild cognitive impairment (discussed in Question 28) and subsequent progression to later stages of AD.

Biological reserve

surplus of capacity of a given organ or system in the body; has to be destroyed before symptoms of the disease occur. For example, studies have shown that initial problems with learning and memory appear in AD after almost 50% of nerve cells in certain parts of the hippocampus are gone.

The concept of **biological reserve** applies to the human brain as it does to many other organs and systems in your body. The biological reserve literally means a surplus of capacity created by a network of nerve cells and their connections; when it's destroyed, disease symptoms occur. Because increased mental activity improves functioning of the neuronal cell network, increased brain activity may help to protect against AD. Intellectual stimulation (use of your brain) appears to bring about greater neuronal connectivity (impulses) and may also influence new neuronal interconnections. A general saying that's often applied to this situation is "Use it or lose it!" Indeed, in older people who remain intellectually active, the risk for developing AD is decreased twofold as compared to age-matched subjects who are not involved in any stimulating thinking activities.

16. Do people with Down syndrome develop AD?

Elizabeth's comment:

My father suffers from AD, so I attended a meeting organized for AD patients' caregivers. After the meeting, I questioned the doctors who delivered a speech about the origin of AD. I told them that I also have a six-year-old son who has diagnosed Down syndrome. I had heard about a relationship between AD and Down syndrome, so I asked, "Does that mean that my son will also develop AD and, if so, when?"

Chromosome

structure carrying DNA-encoding proteins. Humans have 23 pairs of chromosomes.

This question is asked frequently by parents of a child born with Down syndrome. Down syndrome is one of the most common forms of mental retardation and is caused by carrying three (instead of the normal two) copies of **chromosome** 21. Persons with Down syndrome typically have impaired intelligence but may be able to take care of their life needs and in some cases perform a job in a protected environment. Because the gene for the amyloid precursor protein is located on chromosome 21, those with Down syndrome have three instead of two copies of this gene. This increased dosage of the gene leads to overproduction of the amyloid precursor protein and, as a consequence, to an increased amount of amyloid-β. As discussed earlier, amyloid-β is a protein that is deposited in the brain when present in increased amounts, which initiates the symptoms of AD.

Unfortunately, all subjects with Down syndrome will eventually develop AD if they live long enough. AD symptoms among those with Down syndrome show up as a regression of acquired skills (e.g., ability to talk, bathing and toileting skills, ability to cook and shop independently). Although all Down syndrome persons are carrying the same three copies of the chromosome 21 encoding the amyloid precursor protein, the onset of AD symptoms ranges from the mid-thirties to the sixties. We don't fully understand the reasons for this. However, this fact provides strong evidence that AD is a disease caused by many factors and that its onset can be influenced and changed by both genetic (hereditary) and environmental factors.

WHEN SHOULD YOU SUSPECT AD?

17. My memory isn't as good as it used to be. Is this AD?

David's comment:

I'm 66 years old and still work as an accountant for a large insurance company. I've been an accountant for my whole life, and I'm known to be extremely meticulous and precise.

I recently suffered the loss of my brother to cancer. My older sister (who's 75 years old) is in an advanced stage of AD. Recently, I went to the doctor's office complaining about memory difficulties. I told them that I don't feel like my memory is as good as it used to be. Having been an accountant for my whole life, I'm used to remembering numbers after I've just looked at them once. For the past few months, I'm much slower, and I have to check things at work twice or even three times. I've never made a mistake so far, but I've caught myself several times making errors resulting from forgetting things. A week ago, I couldn't find my car on a parking lot in front of a shopping mall in our city. This made me extra anxious. I reminded the doctors that my sister has AD. What a terrible disease! Because of all that's happening to me, I started wondering whether I'm also developing AD and should retire.

Many people feel that their memory becomes less sharp as they get older, and they frequently complain about this to their doctor and family. Most of the concerns involve situations like misplacing objects or not recalling names of people recently met. Minor problems and changes in memory functioning are normal with aging. Part of this age-associated change is not related to memory itself but to a slight decrease of attention with age. When you're putting an object in a given place, you involuntarily record this fact. This function can be easily changed if you're tired, sick, anxious, or distracted and are paying much less attention to what you're doing. As your attention span decreases with age, you might complain often about misplacing such objects as keys, but such events are not symptoms of disease. For comparison, people with true AD frequently do not remember that they were placing keys somewhere and may put them in odd places, such as in the garbage.

Complaints about memory loss in aged persons are very frequent. We always recommend obtaining an opinion from a physician specializing in AD and other dementing diseases. Memory complaints are considered to be a significant sign of disease if they're noticeable to others even though they may not be noticeable to the patient. We're always happy when we can report to our patients that their complaints are those of normal aging and are not symptoms of AD. Frequently, we offer an evaluation after 1 year to assure them that their problem is not progressing.

One of the very first patients evaluated in our center spoke of subjective memory complaints at the age of 71 years. She was given a complete examination, including a battery of neuropsychological tests (discussed in Question 43) that did not suggest the presence of AD. She has been checked yearly since her original visit. Currently, she's been under the care of our center for almost 20 years, and scores on her memory tests are almost unchanged from the original visit, which is the strongest possible proof against AD.

During examination in the office, we frequently ask two questions: "Do you think that your memory is worse than it used to be?" and "Do you think that your memory is worse than your peers'?" Most patients who come in for evaluation of memory complaints but don't have AD answer yes to the first question but—surprisingly—do not confirm that their memory is any worse than their peers' of similar age.

In the case of the patient, David, who commented above, we found during examination that David indeed appeared to have slightly limited attention. He was also moderately depressed by the death of his brother but, on neuropsychological evaluation of his memory and mathematical skills, he did much better than average healthy persons of his age. We offered treatment for his depression and reassured him that we cannot objectively find symptoms of AD. We spent a good deal of time explaining to David that he's also suffering from self-perpetuating anxiety fueled by making small mistakes at work and forgetting where he parked his car. Accepting the making of such small mistakes due to depression and limited concentration is especially difficult for a meticulous person such as David. He came back for his follow-up appointment three months later. His depression lessened with the use of an antidepressant, and he stopped focusing on his small mistakes, which brought him emotional relief. As a result, the pace of his work-related activities came back to normal. (See also Questions 36 and 37 for depression and AD, and Question 39 for medical evaluation of AD patients.).

18. Now that I'm 60, should I worry about developing AD? Can tests predict that?

The major risk factor for developing AD is increasing age, and many people are worried about the prospect of developing this disease, particularly if they've seen a loved one endure the AD process. Currently, no test can predict who will and who will not develop sporadic AD.

AD is by and large a sporadic disease, the beginning of which is influenced by many both changeable and unchangeable risk factors. The unchangeable risk factors are those that cannot be changed at a given point in life and include first-degree relatives with AD, apolipoprotein E genotype (discussed in Question 34), or previous head trauma. These factors greatly increase chances of developing AD but, even if they exist, you still have a good chance of not developing AD. In addition, other risk factors can be changed, thereby decreasing your chance of developing AD: elevated cholesterol, continually elevated blood pressure, diabetes, and an elevated level of homocysteine (discussed in Question 35). You should focus on early detection and correction of these disorders as part of routine health care maintenance during middle and advanced age.

For the much less common form of AD—early-onset familial AD—genetic testing (discussed in Question 45) for mutations (defects) in the presenilin 1, presenilin 2, and APP genes is available. Early-onset familial AD begins with dementia typically *before* the age of 60. For individuals with a familial AD–associated alteration in one of these genes, the chances of developing AD are close to 100%, if they live long enough. The typical age of onset of disease with each of these changes varies and, in some cases, a particular mutation may be associated with a wide range of disease severity and onset. Whether undergoing this type of genetic testing is appropriate for you and what the results mean are issues best discussed with a knowledgeable physician.

19. Will diabetes and high blood pressure raise my risk of developing AD?

Unfortunately, the answer to that question is bad news. Large **epidemiological studies** (studies examining occurrence of a given disease in large populations and its coexistence with other conditions) have shown that

Epidemiological studies

studies aiming to determine frequency of given diseases in the population and their association with such factors as age and gender or with other diseases (e.g., diabetes, elevated cholesterol, or cancer).

people who have elevated blood pressure and diabetes have a severalfold increased risk for dementia, including AD. The direct mechanism of how elevated blood pressure and glucose (blood sugar) levels may influence AD remains to be explained. Hypertension and diabetes are also risk factors for vascular dementia (discussed in Question 46). The silver lining is that both these conditions currently can be easily controlled. This may require life-long use of pills and certain changes in your lifestyle (e.g., cutting down on sugar and salt, losing weight), but current medical science has the resources to successfully maintain your blood sugar and pressure levels within the proper range. A number of well-tolerated medications for both conditions are available on the market. People at risk have to remain under the constant care of a physician, but the potential benefit is great: significant lowering of your chance of developing stroke, heart attack, and dementia.

20. Does elevated cholesterol increase my risk of developing AD?

People whose cholesterol was elevated during mid-life tend to develop AD more frequently than those whose cholesterol level was normal.

A continuing elevated level of cholesterol is a well-known risk factor for heart disease and stroke (discussed in Question 12). Recent studies have demonstrated that elevated cholesterol in the forties and fifties is a strong risk factor for developing sporadic AD after the age of 65. As we mentioned, AD starts with the buildup of amyloid-β in the brain many years before the onset of memory symptoms. Many research experiments have demonstrated that an elevated cholesterol level in the blood increases amyloid-β production and allows it to leave deposits. People whose cholesterol was elevated during midlife tend to

develop AD more frequently than those whose cholesterol level was normal. These studies also showed that
an elevation of cholesterol severe enough to increase
the risk for AD does not have to be great. According
to current standards of medical practice, the acceptable
upper level of total cholesterol is 200 mg/dL. A steady
elevation of cholesterol in the range 220 to 250 mg/dL
was enough to change the odds for the onset of AD.
Besides causing a direct impact on amyloid-β production and buildup, a high cholesterol level is a strong
risk factor for stroke, occlusion (clogging) of arteries,
and vascular dementia (all discussed in Question 28).
These factors can add to cognitive deficit produced by
AD and hasten the rate of AD progression (discussed
in Question 31). Therefore, maintaining a normal cholesterol level throughout life is preferable and can be
benefit you in both your mental and your cardiovascular (heart and blood) health.

Why do people have elevated cholesterol? In some, it's
a result of diet containing a high amount of fat from
meat. Increased intake of these unhealthy fats directly
figures in an increased chance for AD, heart attack,
and stroke. You can lower your cholesterol by daily
exercise and by maintaining a diet containing a large
amount of fibers, fruit, vegetables, and unsaturated
fatty acids (from fish) and also by decreasing the
amount of **saturated fatty acids** from meat. You can
manage the latter either by decreasing the total
amount of meat you consume or by switching to lean
meat products or to poultry. Limiting the number of
eggs (especially yolks) and amount of ice cream,
chocolate, and sugary snacks, may improve your cholesterol balance as well. In many people, these simple

Saturated fatty acids

elements abundant
in red meat (e.g.,
pork or beef).
Increased intake of
saturated fatty acids
is associated with
elevated risk of
atherosclerosis and,
as a consequence,
occurrence of stroke
or heart attack.

measures are enough to bring a balance to the cholesterol metabolism. Unfortunately, in others a primary-care physician has to recommend a cholesterol-lowering treatment.

Statins

drugs lowering cholesterol levels and thereby reducing risk of heart attack and stroke. Clinical studies designed to determine whether they may also slow the course of AD are ongoing.

Nowadays, the class of drugs most frequently prescribed to lower cholesterol are **statins**. These drugs are simple to use (once a day before bedtime) and have very few side effects. The following statins are available in the U.S. market: atorvastatin (Lipitor); fluvastatin (Lescol); lovastatin (Mevacor); pravastatin (Pravachol); and simvastatin (Zocor). All these drugs work in a similar way and should be prescribed by a physician who will select the best drug for you and will monitor the treatment effect. During treatment with statins, liver function test results must be checked regularly. Recommended cholesterol levels for starting anticholesterol treatment, provided that changes in your diet produced no satisfactory decrease, are as follows: total cholesterol above 200 mg/dL, LDL fraction above 130 mg/dL, triglyceride fraction above 160 mg/dL, or HDL fraction (also called a "good cholesterol") below 40 mg/dL. Remember: The normal level of cholesterol, not statins per se, reduces your risk for sporadic AD, heart attack, and stroke.

SYMPTOMS

21. What are the first symptoms of AD?

The human mind is extremely complicated, so disease affecting the mind may produce a wide variety of symptoms. AD may emerge with a large variety of signs but, in the majority of cases, the picture is dominated by a failing in learning and memory. Many people notice with advancing age that their memory is not as good as it used to be (discussed in Question 17); they more frequently misplace things or they cannot find the right word when they speak. These signs may be only minor failings brought on by normal aging, but they also may be early symptoms of AD. The key issues in separating minor age-related problems from true symptoms of the disease is checking to see whether these symptoms are noticeable to other people, actively interfere with your daily activities or job performance, and can be seen during examinations in a doctor's office or through **neuropsychological testing** (discussed in Question 43). Below is a list of early signs associated with AD.

Neuropsychological testing

series of tests measuring various intellectual functions (e.g., memory, language, intelligence, judgment, problem solving, spatial orientation, and others) and used in AD to detect and measure deficits in various areas of cognition and memory in particular.

- *Difficulties with remembering things and learning:* As was emphasized, easily forgetting recently learned information (discussed in Question 9) is the most characteristic sign of AD. Although it's normal sometimes to forget names, telephone numbers, or even appointments, in AD this is more frequent and concerns more vital facts, such as missing an important job meeting that could have serious results. Also, those suffering from AD frequently do not have awareness that they have forgotten something important; that's not the case with normally cognitive individuals. Learning new job-related tasks comes to AD patients with great difficulty and is sometimes almost impossible.
- *Misplacing things:* Almost everyone will temporarily misplace a key or a wallet. Frequently, a distraction will cause this so that the action could not be properly recorded. People with AD often place objects in a place they would not normally belong, say, a toothbrush in a desk drawer or a key in a refrigerator.

• *Language problems:* The problem of finding the right words may happen to any one of us, especially when we're tired or under stress. This usually affects less commonly used words, but a normal person can swiftly find synonyms so that speech is fluent. In those with AD, loss of word choice may be noticeable several times a day, and AD patients have difficulties with finding a synonym as well. Also, they can forget more commonly used words, and understanding their speech can be difficult. Those who cannot find a comb may ask for "a thing for hair." In addition, AD patients may not understand more sophisticated and less frequently used words or may make errors in substituting words that sound similar but have different meanings, thus making their speech confusing to others.

• *Disorientation as to place and time:* One of the most frequent concerns is that we might lose a car in a parking lot from time to time. This obviously is an embarrassing incident but usually is related to distraction and not paying attention when parking, especially when nothing notable stands out on the parking lot. People with AD are frequently lost in an unfamiliar neighborhood and even on their own street, and they do not know how to get back home (discussed in Questions 84 and 85). Typically, an AD patient would get lost in the vicinity where the car was parked and have no memory of even coming there by car, rather than searching the parking lot for the missing vehicle.

AD patients may have difficulties with recording time and therefore may not give a correct date.

Such people may forget the day of the week, especially when there is little to make a distinction between the days (e.g., when on vacation or in a hospital). A normal person is usually aware of the approximate time of day. AD patients may have difficulties with recording time and therefore may not give a correct date. Even if the correct date is given to them, they may not remember it when asked some time later. AD patients also have difficulty in stating the approximate time of day without looking at their watch.

- *Decrease in judgment:* An AD-caused problem of judgment about simple matters is usually obvious to others. This includes such situations as dressing incorrectly for outdoor weather or spending large amounts of money for unneeded things or services. AD patients also may be easily persuaded by various people to pay large amounts of money for unneeded, poor-quality home improvements or to give away large sums for charities, in contrast to their prior behavior.

- *Decreased problem-solving skills:* AD patients have difficulties with balancing a checkbook or with organizing things (e.g., dinner for a large number of people). They may be overwhelmed by shopping for an unusually large number of guests, calculating how many pieces of silverware may be needed, or how to seat people around the table.

- *Difficulty with familiar tasks:* Some tasks are so familiar that we don't think about them: preparing meals, using household appliances, or participating in a lifelong hobby. An AD patient, on the contrary, may perform such simple activities with increasing difficulty and frequently may leave them unfinished.

- *Loss of initiative:* Frequently, people with AD display loss of initiative (willpower) and spontaneity (natural impulse). They may slowly withdraw from work obligations, be increasingly less active during family meetings, or stop participating in social events. They may spend time very passively on tasks with low productivity.

- *Changes in mood or behavior:* Changes in mood or behavior may happen without control and more often than is seen in normal people. Rapid swings from calm to tears or from calm to anger may occur for no apparent reason.

- *Personality changes:* Although personality may slightly alter with age, people with AD may demonstrate profound changes (e.g., becoming extremely suspicious, greedy or unreasonably generous, fearful, or aggressive). They frequently may become very dependent on a family member.

22. How do the symptoms of AD evolve over time?

AD is a disease that slowly advances over a number of years. Extensive experience gathered by scientists and physicians has shown that, in the majority of cases, AD progresses in an organized fashion from one stage to the next. The **global deterioration scale** is one instrument often used by physicians to follow the progress of AD. This scale has seven stages that chart the progression of AD from normal to very advanced dementia.

Global deterioration scale

scale used by physicians to measure progression of AD.

Stage 1: Normal

Stage 1 describes any person, at any age, who is free of subjective (personal) or objective complaints (those obvious to physician and others) regarding memory function or other aspects of the mind. The person in stage one is also free of personality, mood, and behavior changes.

Stage 2: Benign aged forgetfulness

Stage 2 clusters people who feel that their memory is not functioning as it used to (discussed in Question 17). These concerns in most cases arise because, with advancing age, they can no longer recall names as well as they could 5 or 10 years ago. They are also very frequently convinced that they can no longer recall where they have placed such things as keys and sunglasses. They may also experience personal difficulties with concentration and finding the correct word while speaking. All these problems remain subjective and are not noticed by family, friends, or coworkers or during examination by a physician.

Stage 3: Mild cognitive impairment

In stage 3 as charted by the global deterioration scale, others can notice limits in learning and making new memories that can be measured in clinical testing. Patients show a decreased ability to remember names when introduced to new people, noticeably repeat queries, retain little material when they read a passage or watch television, frequently misplace valuable objects, and show a decline in their ability to plan and organize. Family and associates notice word- and name-finding problems. All these deficits result in a decreased performance at work and in more difficulties in the activities of daily living. People in this stage no longer can master or learn such new skills as computer skills. Increased anxiety is common. Frequently, professionally active patients are forced to retire.

Stage 3 lasts on average 7 years. The diagnosis is usually made when this stage has progressed midway, but if AD patients haven't been called on to perform complex social or occupational tasks, symptoms may not become evident to family members or friends or even to such patients. By the end of this stage, a confident diagnosis of early-stage AD can be made in most (but not all) patients.

Stage 4: Mild AD

In stage 4, a memory deficit becomes more evident. AD patients may not recall many major events, such as holidays, social parties, or visits to relatives. They frequently make mistakes in recalling the day of the week, the month, or a season. They're able, however, to give their address correctly, name the head of state, or describe outdoor weather conditions. Mathematical skills are affected; therefore, patients in this stage frequently cannot balance a check book and may have difficulties with paying bills. Their capacity to perform complex tasks (e.g., shopping for food or preparing meals for the family) gradually becomes impaired.

Such patients also become less emotionally responsive than previously, are socially withdrawn, and frequently depend on others, especially when they cannot cope with a new situation. For example, when asked about something, they may answer "I don't remember, but my wife would know," or in a restaurant, they depend on others to order their food. This stage lasts, on average, 2 years.

Stage 5: Moderate AD

In stage 5, the memory deficit progresses and involves not only current events but major events from the past. Patients may not be able to give their current address, telephone number, or year, or the name of the current president. They're not able to recall the name of the college or school from which they graduated. They usually retain substantial knowledge about themselves and know the names of their spouse and children.

Arithmetic is severely impaired. Stage 5 patients can't count backward from 40 by 4s or from 20 by 2s. The cognitive (intellectual) deficit at this stage is so great that accident-free survival is impossible if such patients are left without help. Patients can no longer manage in the absence of someone to assist in providing meals and ensure that their rent and utilities are paid. This stage lasts approximately between 1 year to 18 months.

Stage 6: Moderately severe AD

At stage 6, AD patients gradually lose their ability to perform basic activities of daily living. One of the first signs of this stage is loss of the ability to choose the right clothes and put them on properly. For example, patients in this stage may have difficulties in putting an arm in the correct sleeve, or they may be dressing backward or in the wrong order (discussed in Question 78). Patients also lose their ability to bathe independently (discussed in Question 81). One of the earliest signs of a bathing deficit is difficulty in adjusting the water temperature. Losing bathing skills frequently goes hand in hand with other deficits in daily hygiene, such as brushing teeth or combing hair (discussed in Question 81).

As the disease progresses, stage 6 patients no longer can manage the mechanics of toileting properly. Not flushing the toilet or misplacing toilet tissue is common. This is followed by incontinence: first urinary, then bowel incontinence (discussed in Question 83). Sleep disturbances are also common. Throughout this stage, patients remember their name but frequently are mistaken about names of their close family members. Not uncommonly, such patients confuse their spouse with a deceased parent. Calculation (figuring) is impaired to the point that patients cannot count backward from 10 by 1's. Limits of speech become obvious. Neologisms (when patients make up new words) and stuttering render their speech difficult to understand.

Family and caregivers may notice significant changes in personality and disturbances in behavior (discussed in Question 76). Some patients may become suspicious or **delusional** (e.g., believing that a spouse is an impostor). **Hallucinations** (seeing or hearing things that are not real) or compulsive or repetitive behaviors (e.g., paper shredding) may become frequent (discussed in Questions 72 and 73). Patients go through this stage for perhaps 2 to 2.5 years.

Stage 7: Severe (end-stage) AD

In stage 7, patients require continuous assistance with basic activities. Speech becomes severely impaired, and language may be limited to only several understandable words. Eventually, such patients lose their ability to speak. They show increasing difficulties with independent walking (discussed in Question 24). First they may require more and more assistance, and finally they are confined to a wheelchair or bed. As the disease progresses, patients lose their ability to sit independently and then to smile. In this, the final stage, they are

Delusions

false beliefs not shared by others. They tend to be maintained firmly even if they don't agree with reality and even if they are strongly contradicted by others.

Hallucinations

false notions of nonexisting objects or happenings. They may affect all senses; therefore, types include visual hallucination (seeing nonexisting things), sensory hallucination (feeling touch when nothing is touching), or auditory hallucination (hearing nonexisting voices).

unable to hold up their head independently, and they develop prolonged spasms, called contractions, in their extremities. It usually takes 5 years for a patient to progress to this very end stage. With intensive nursing and medical care, patients are able to survive in this final stage of AD for several years.

23. Is the course of AD always the same?

The course of AD described here is true for most AD patients, with multiple disease stages following one another and with progressing memory impairment (failure) a major feature. Rarely, AD may start as a deficit in judgment, making plans, and solving problems or with an inability to process visual information. In the latter situation, patients see a picture but cannot appreciate its meaning. In such cases, memory first is somewhat or partially preserved. With time, such patient's symptoms progress to global dementia (discussed in Questions 28 and 29), as in AD with a more classic course. What has to be emphasized here is that in these (less common) cases, the diagnosis of AD was made only after a patient's death. The clinical course of such cases can resemble other forms of dementias (e.g., **frontotemporal dementia**, discussed in Question 28).

Another frequent occurrence is that a patient may have more than one type of brain pathology (disease) combined, such as AD and vascular dementia or AD and Parkinson's disease (discussed in Question 28). Some one-third of AD patients also experience either a stroke or another kind of vascular brain impairment. These additional factors may change the course of AD, with some symptoms appearing in stages of the

Frontotemporal dementia
neurodegenerative disease much rarer than AD and also leading to dementia.

Some one-third of AD patients also experience either a stroke or another kind of vascular brain impairment.

disease when they normally are not observed. For example, for somebody who suffers from Parkinson's disease, walking may be a disability in much earlier stages of AD, whereas a stroke may affect the ability to walk or speak in those whose memory is fairly good.

24. Can AD impair gait?

The ability to walk is spared in AD until the late stages of disease. AD patients may not be able to remember things and might have significant speech difficulties, but at the same time they may be able to walk. Their motor skills, such as in handling objects, may not be impaired. As a rule, when difficulty with walking precedes dementia or accompanies cognitive deficit from the beginning, other conditions are much more likely: vascular dementia, Parkinson's disease, Lewy body dementia, **normal-pressure hydrocephalus**, progressive supranuclear palsy, or **Huntington's disease**. Those who experience strokes often have problems either with weakness or with coordination, making ambulation (walking) difficult. If patients with dementia have a walking difficulty early in the course of their AD, another diagnosis should be considered besides AD; there may be another problem that is responsible for the dementia and gait problem or exists together with AD.

Normal-pressure hydrocephalus

disease associated with excess of cerebrospinal fluid and seen in progressing problems with walking, urinary continence, and eventually dementia.

Huntington's disease

inherited neurodegenerative disease associated with difficulty in controlling "dance-like" movements and eventually with dementia.

25. Is the sense of smell affected by AD?

Yes, a deficit in the sense of smell is very common among AD patients. The part of the brain responsible for processing odors lies very close to your hippocampus (memory center). Like the hippocampus, it is very prone to the AD disease process. The sense of smell can be affected in AD very early in the course of the disease. Research has also shown that otherwise healthy elderly people who have an affected sense of smell more frequently develop AD than do those with a good sense of smell. Although this fact was very well known for many years, it is difficult to judge on the basis of the sense of smell alone who will and who will not develop AD. Impairment in the sense of smell is very unspecific and may be related to many local conditions (e.g., sinus disease, allergies, medications, smoking, nasal surgery, a cold, or an overuse of nasal drops).

Many people have a poor sense of smell to begin with and, in all individuals, the sense of smell gets blunted with age. Studies have also shown that older people with a good sense of smell are not free from the risk of developing AD. Therefore, an impaired ability to pick up various scents should not be a reason for increased fear of oncoming disease. One caregiver in our practice, whose mother died recently of AD, reported her lack of any sense of smell for more than 10 years. The caregiver worried that she was developing AD and that a familial form might be present in her family. In such a middle-aged person with normally functioning memory, the risk of other disease destroying the sense of smell overshadows the possibility of AD, especially if symptoms are present for more than 10 years without developing any cognitive loss. In this situation, it's advisable to refer this person to see an ear, nose, and throat specialist (**otolaryngologist**) to determine a cause or causes contributing to the loss of a sense of smell.

Otolaryngologist
doctor specializing in treating ear, nose, and throat diseases.

26. Are AD patients aware of memory loss?

Luckily, we're able to make a more benign (less harmful) diagnosis in many patients who come to our office for evaluation of memory complaints: normal aging-related forgetfulness, depression, or anxiety. Strikingly, in many true AD patients, memory and other intellectual problems may go unnoticed for a long time, even until a patient advances to stage four (discussed in Question 22). This frequently happens in people who are retired and are not required to perform challenging social tasks and who have family support for activities of daily living. As a result, symptoms of AD remain hidden until the moment they encounter a more challenging situation. In many situations, both patients and their families are not overly concerned. The memory deficiency is accepted as something naturally associated with aging. In addition, such people frequently use denial as a mechanism of defense, and they may actively displace from their minds the possibility of AD. An example is seen in the story of one patient who came to our office in stage four of the global deterioration scale.

Sylvia's comment:

I noticed that my father increasingly forgets more and more things regarding daily living matters. He's 72 years old, and he retired at the age of 65 but worked part-time till he was 68. After my mom passed away nine years ago due to breast cancer, he had an episode of grief but never symptoms of depression. He lives alone a few blocks away from our home and sometime helps us with our two boys, picking them up after school and driving them to various after-

school activities, especially when my husband is on a business trip and I have to stay longer at work. I admit I wouldn't notice anything, but my younger son, who's six years old, told me that grandpa again forgot when he had to drive him one afternoon. A month later, I received a call from my son's karate coach that somebody should have picked him up after the practice. I drove and picked my son up but was frankly surprised because I'd asked my father to do so a day before and reminded him about this over the phone during lunchtime the same day. When I called him afterward, he was regretful and surprised that he could forget it. From this time on, I paid a little more attention to his household, and I noticed on his desk a few unpaid bills and bounced checks. There were also returned checks which he hadn't signed. He never admitted these things were happening to him. He was always punctual and accurate. He spent most of his professional life as a bank officer. Finances and math were his domain.

In the situation she described, the daughter finally noticed and realized that her father's behavior was abnormal, which prompted medical evaluation and making the correct diagnosis. In certain situations, however, families are subconsciously in denial and accept the cognitive decline in parents or grandparents as a part of normal aging until much later stages of the disease. It's usually only a matter of time until a significant problem occurs, such as being lost in unfamiliar surroundings or being agitated because of a minor infection or medical illness. This usually creates a need for making the correct diagnosis and for the family to accept the fact that their beloved one suffers from AD. The currently increased consciousness regarding AD has led to making more accurate diagnoses earlier.

In certain situations, families are subconsciously in denial and accept the cognitive decline in parents or grandparents as a part of normal aging until much later stages of the disease.

IT'S DEMENTIA, BUT IS IT AD? THE DIAGNOSIS DILEMMA

27. How reliable is a clinical diagnosis of AD?

Currently, only an examination of the brain after death can give a certain diagnosis of AD. In most situations, however, the clinical diagnosis made by a neurologist (a doctor specializing in treatment of nervous system diseases) is accurate. The process of making the diagnosis is based on recognition of a pattern of cognitive deficit, with prominent memory symptoms from the beginning; normal balance, gait, and movements at early stages; and a lack of abnormalities on **magnetic resonance imaging** (MRI) other than shrinking of the hippocampus (Figure 6). Equally important is to rule out treatable conditions producing dementia, such as depression, **hypothyroidism**, or vitamin B_{12} deficiency. A diagnosis of probable AD means that the

Magnetic resonance imaging

method of taking pictures of living brains that is used by doctors to diagnose and follow up brain disease (e.g., AD) and is based on the use of a high-power magnetic field.

Hypothyroidism

abnormally low function of the thyroid gland associated with slow metabolism, lower heart rate, cold intolerance, leg edema, and (in older people) symptoms of dementia.

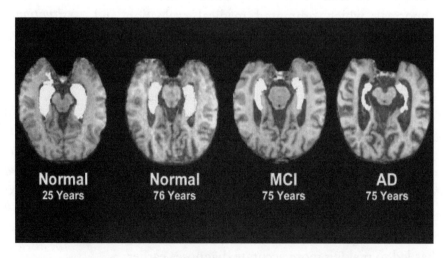

Figure 6 **Magnetic resonance imaging (MRI) scans showing shrinkage of the hippocampus (the memory and learning center shown in red) in the mild cognitive impairment (MCI) and in AD. (Image courtesy of Dr. Mony DeLeon, New York University.)**

physician has ruled out all other disorders that may be causing dementia and has come to the conclusion that the symptoms are most likely the result of AD. A comparison between a physician's diagnosis of probable AD and autopsy results shows that physicians are 90% correct when the clinical evaluations are done by experienced specialists. In rare cases, however, either AD has an unusual course, mimicking other forms of dementia, or it coexists with other neurodegenerative (nerve cell–damaging) illness.

28. What other brain diseases cause dementia?

Besides AD, many other brain diseases cause dementia. However, AD is the most frequent cause of dementia. The dementia can also be a consequence of strokes, brain inflammation, toxins, or tumors. Diseases leading to dementia other than AD are briefly described in this and following questions, in order of decreasing frequency. We focus on neurodegenerative disorders other than AD. Together they are five to seven times less common than AD.

- *Frontotemporal dementia*: After AD, frontotemporal dementia is the third most frequent neurodegenerative disease leading to dementia. It was originally known as *Pick's disease*. The disease affects mainly nerve cells of the frontal and temporal lobes of the brain. The clinical picture shows mainly the inability to make long-term plans, incorrect social behavior, impaired impulse control (e.g., inability to control spending or appetite), and lack of sexual control. The disease also brings loss of personal awareness and neglect of hygiene and grooming (discussed in Question 81). One of the proteins involved in the failure of neural cells in frontotemporal dementia is the tau protein (discussed in Question 7). That's the same protein involved in the formation of neurofibrillary tangles, which attribute to death of neural cells in AD. In rare familial cases, the disease can be caused by a mutation in the tau protein. Unlike AD, amyloid-β deposits are absent in this disorder.

Lewy-body dementia

form of dementia caused by degeneration of nerve cells that accumulate as structures called Lewy bodies made up of α-synuclein.

α-synuclein

protein that builds up in excessive amounts in nerve cells in Parkinson's disease and Lewy-body dementia. Accumulation of α-synuclein in nerve cells causes Lewy bodies. Accumulation of α-synuclein in nerve cells leads to their dysfunction and death.

Substantia nigra

part of the brain severely affected in Parkinson's disease, causing tremor, slow movements, and disability in walking.

- *Lewy-body dementia*: **Lewy-body dementia** is caused by a disorder of a protein called a α-synuclein, which leads to death of neurons (nerve cells) in the brain cortex and other structures as the **substantia nigra**. In this disease, α-synuclein builds up within neurons and forms ball-like structures called *Lewy bodies*. This type of dementia is accompanied by frequent agitation and visual hallucinations (discussed in Questions 69 and 72). It is the second most common neurodegenerative disease causing dementia after AD.

- *Parkinson's disease–related dementia*: Parkinson's disease is a dysfunction of the movement-controlling system, resulting in slowing of movements and tremors of the hands, feet, and (sometimes) head. As the disease progresses, keeping balance and walking become a problem (discussed in Question 24). Many patients who reach the advanced stage of this disease show symptoms of cognitive problems. Parkinson's disease is also related to a disorder of α-synuclein, causing it to build up in nerve cells and form Lewy bodies (as discussed here). In rare familial cases, mutations are found in the α-synuclein protein, which cause it to form Lewy bodies more easily. However, most cases of Parkinson's disease (e.g., AD) are sporadic, and we don't know what causes the formation of Lewy bodies. In Parkinson's disease, Lewy bodies are found just in the substantia nigra, a deep part of the brain important in the control of your movements.

- *Huntington's disease*: Huntington's disease is a purely genetic disease seen in excess of movements (patients appear to be dancing) and dementia. The onset of the disease varies from the thirties to the seventies. It is caused by a mutation in the specific protein called Huntington.

- *Corticobasal ganglionic degeneration*: **Corticobasal ganglionic degeneration**, a form of dementia, is fairly rare and at first appears as a disorder that causes asymmetrical (uneven) abnormal movement. Patients report clumsiness, loss of dexterity, and a lack of sensation, usually in one hand. Later on, problems in performing certain tasks with affected limbs (e.g., combing hair or cutting bread) become evident, although muscle strength in the affected limb is preserved. This symptom is called **apraxia**, which means an inability to perform a known task, even though the strength of the limb is normal. In addition to the problems with movement, it causes a progressive cognitive (intellectual) failure.

- *Progressive supranuclear palsy*: **Progressive supranuclear palsy**, another rare form of dementia, exhibits some symptoms similar to those seen in Parkinson's disease. As in Parkinson's disease, movements of extremities are slow, but usually those affected don't experience tremors. Unlike true Parkinson's disease, balance problems and frequent falls are present from the beginning of the disease, as is significant dementia. The most typical feature of this condition is an inability to look down. When asked, patients cannot willingly turn their eyes downward. This disease almost never exists in subjects younger than age 50.

Corticobasal ganglionic degeneration
rare form of neuro-degenerative disease leading to dementia and motor dysfunction.

Apraxia
inability to perform certain tasks (e.g., cutting bread, waving good-bye) despite preservation of strength. The problem is usually associated with a neurodegenerative disease and related to losing ability to execute once-learned tasks.

Progressive supranuclear palsy
rare form of neuro-degenerative disease resembling Parkinson's disease but, unlike Parkinson's disease, producing problems with directing gaze downward, frequent falls, and eventual severe problems with swallowing.

**Primary progres-
sive aphasia**

rare form of neuro-
degenerative disease
leading to dementia
in which the primary
and leading problem
is associated with
language dys-
function.

*Many times,
as patients
age, they have
more than one
disease process
taking place in
their brains.*

Gastritis

inflammation of the
stomach.

• *Primary progressive aphasia*: **Primary progressive aphasia**, a rare form of dementia, has a gradual onset and at the beginning involves only language problems. This is seen as a slowly progressing difficulty with remembering correct words and understanding more difficult phrases. Gradually, sentences become less complete and are shortened to just a few words. In the final stage, affected patients' language is limited to only several words. Eventually, such patients become mute and do not respond to voice at all.

Often these diseases exist together with some degree of AD symptoms, which can also contribute to cognitive limitations. Many times, as patients age, they have more than one disease process taking place in their brains. Especially among Parkinson's disease patients, a combination of AD or Lewy-body disease symptoms very frequently causes dementia. Researchers do not understand the routes of all these neurodegenerative (nerve cell–damaging) diseases causing dementia and of those causing AD. Unfortunately, as in AD, there is no effective treatment for any of them currently.

29. Are any types of dementia reversible?

Yes, some are. Therefore, when evaluating a patient for AD, a neurologist has to exclude those types of disorders. Poisons, infections, or lack of certain types of vitamins or hormones may cause symptoms of dementia that can be reversed by treatment. Deficiency of vitamin B_{12} is such an example. This condition may occur in people who have had certain types of extensive gastrointestinal surgery, after which their intake of vitamin B_{12} is limited. Other people may have a rare form of **gastritis**, also limiting their supply of B_{12}. Symptoms of vitamin B_{12} deficiency have an almost unnoticed onset and a slow course, such as those of AD. The diagnosis of this type of dementia can be made by checking the level of vitamin B_{12} in the blood.

Frequently in older people, owing to changes in their **metabolism**, their level of vitamin B_{12} is on the low side of the normal range. In such a situation, the doctor can check their level of **methylmalonic acid**. An elevation of methylmalonic acid is seen with an unnoticed type of vitamin B_{12} deficit. Because lack of vitamin B_{12} can add to cognitive problems caused by the AD process, a doctor should check the levels of vitamin B_{12} and methylmalonic acid when a patient is evaluated for dementia.

Metabolism

all chemical reactions taking place in a living organism.

Methylmalonic acid

molecule associated with metabolism of vitamin B_{12}. Measurement of its level is a more sensitive marker of vitamin B_{12} deficiency, the level of vitamin B_{12} itself.

Treatment includes giving patients vitamin B_{12} preparations. If vitamin B_{12} deficiency is caused by interrupted intake from the intestine because of gastrointestinal disease, vitamin B_{12} can be administered by injection into muscles.

Another cause of reversible dementia is an incomplete production of **thyroid hormones**. In the typical form of thyroid deficiency, patients have such symptoms as obesity, cold intolerance, a slow heart rate, dry skin, and decreased endurance for physical exercise. This may be followed by damage to their cognitive function. The condition can be reversed by giving such patients thyroid hormones in the form of pills.

Thyroid hormones

hormones secreted by thyroid gland and essential for maintaining proper metabolism of the body. Their deficiency may cause symptoms of dementia (among other symptoms) in the elderly.

Elderly individuals may also experience a partially blocked thyroid function owing to the aging process.

In such a situation, thyroid deficiency rarely itself causes the symptoms of dementia. Just as with low levels of vitamin B_{12}, this minor deficiency can contribute to the mental slowness caused primarily by AD, vascular dementia (discussed in Question 30), or other types of dementing illness. Therefore, normal clinical practice is to check the level of thyroid hormones in evaluating for dementia. If it is below normal, treatment that includes taking daily oral doses of thyroid hormones can be started. To avoid side effects (e.g., **cardiac arrhythmia**), the desired dosage is achieved over a few weeks to months. The response to treatment can be easily checked by retesting the levels of thyroid hormones while on medications.

Cardiac arrhythmia
heart rate abnormality.

Examples of infections causing dementia are acquired immunodeficiency syndrome (AIDS), syphilis, and fungal meningitis. AIDS is caused by infection with the human immunodeficiency virus (HIV), which can be passed on by sexual contact, or exposure to hypodermic needles or blood contaminated with HIV. Both AIDS and syphilis can affect the brain secretly years after actual infection takes place, and the onset of brain disease may go undetected. Therefore, many physicians recommend checking for syphilis and HIV infection if there is any possibility of exposure. If detected early by blood tests, progression of dementia due to syphilis can be halted. Dementia due to syphilis infection was once common; this type of dementia is extremely rare nowadays. Adequate treatment of HIV infection can greatly reduce the cases of brain complications.

Meningitis
inflammation of the membranes surrounding and protecting the brain; can be caused by bacteria or fungus).

Fungal meningitis produces cognitive deficit with headache and, frequently, paralysis of some nerves. If detected early in the infection, the condition can be reversed with antibiotics.

30. What is vascular dementia?

Vascular dementia is the second most common form of dementia, surpassed only by AD itself. In this type of dementia, nerve cells and connections between them are damaged as a result of closure of large or small arteries supplying your brain with blood; that in turn deprives nerve cells of oxygen and nutrients. Vascular dementia may be seen in several distinctly different ways, depending on whether large or small or both types of arteries are closed.

Multi-infarct dementia is a subtype of vascular dementia in which damage to the brain occurs as a result of multiple infarcts, also called ischemic strokes. These infarcts or ischemic strokes almost always result from closing off of one of the main brain arteries. The word "multi" means that more than one infarct occurs, usually over a period of months to years. Therefore, multi-infarct dementia has a stepwise course. The resulting mental deficit gets worse with each subsequent infarct and clearly depends on the size of infarctions, their number, and the site of infarctions in the brain. Remember that the brain is a highly specialized organ (discussed in Question 9). For example, the first infarct may strike the area of brain responsible for language, the second (happening months to years later) may hit the area responsible for mathematical skills, and the third may damage an area involved in the memory process. Some degree of improvement is possible between strokes. Also unlike AD, vascular dementia is often associated with motor weakness and imbalance.

Multi-infarct dementia

dementia resulting from numerous and repetitive strokes.

Closing off of numerous small vessels produces a quite distinct picture of vascular dementia. These small vessels are ultimate branches of large arteries that run down from the brain surface and provide nutrients and oxygen to deeply lying structures, including the white matter of your brain. The white matter is literally a buildup of long connections wiring particular nerve cells. In other words, closing off these small vessels leads to disruption of communication between neural cells. These small vessels are very sensitive to damage caused by lengthy and untreated elevated blood pressure and diabetes (discussed in Question 19), elevated cholesterol (discussed in Question 20), and smoking. Unlike those of multiinfarct dementia, symptoms of dementia resulting from small-vessel disease begin almost unnoticed and progress slowly, just as in AD, but rarely start with outstanding memory complaints. Magnetic resonance imaging (MRI) can easily weigh the extent of brain damage from small-vessel disease. Originally, small-vessel ischemic (blood-deprived) brain disease caused by uncontrolled, elevated blood pressure was described by a German physician, Otto Binswanger, at the end of the nineteenth century; therefore, this form of vascular dementia is frequently called **Binswanger's disease**.

Binswanger's disease

form of vascular dementia caused by closing off small vessels supplying the white matter of the brain.

The small-vessel disease is a slow, ongoing process. Sudden closure of a small artery may also happen, resulting in a **lacunar infarction**, which is a small infarction with a size usually less than 1 cm. Often, when a lacunar infarction happens, it may go unnoticed. Rarely, if a lacunar infarct is located within an important brain region, it may produce a major intellectual deficit similar to that observed with major strokes.

Lacunar infarction

small brain infarction or stroke (less than 10 mm).

Small-vessel disease with or without lacunar infarcts more frequently causes a vascular dementia than does multiinfarct dementia. Most patients suffering from multiinfarct dementia will have some degree of small-vessel disease, but the opposite is uncommon.

Common risk factors for large strokes (causing multi-infarct dementia) and small-vessel disease include **hypertension**, **hypercholesterolemia**, diabetes, and smoking. Large infarcts may also result from an **embolism** related to a heart disease. This occurs when a blood clot originating from a diseased heart flows with the bloodstream to one of the major arteries supplying the brain and closes the artery off, depriving part of the brain from oxygen and nutrients. Currently, no treatment exists for damage from ischemia that has already taken place. Therefore, prevention of stroke is a key issue (discussed in Question 12). Primary prevention identifies stroke risk factors (e.g., elevated blood pressure, diabetes, elevated cholesterol) and includes their forceful treatment. Secondary prevention gives stroke-preventing medications to people who have had a stroke in the past. The most basic stroke prevention medication is a small dose of aspirin taken daily. Some people, especially these suffering from a heart condition, have to take a blood thinner (Coumadin).

31. What is mild cognitive impairment?

Mild cognitive impairment is a diagnosis assigned to mild but noticeable memory problems. People with mild cognitive impairment (damage) have an isolated difficulty in learning and memorizing new things while other aspects of their intellect are functioning

Hypertension
elevated blood pressure occurring in every fourth person after age 50 and forming a significant risk factor for stroke and heart attack if untreated.

Hypercholester-olemia
elevated level of cholesterol due to increased cholesterol intake, inherited predisposition, or both. Hypercholesterolemia is a risk factor for heart attack, stroke, and AD.

Embolism
blood clot or other material (e.g., fat) that travels with the bloodstream and can lodge in an artery too small to allow it to pass. An embolus lodging in the brain artery may cause a stroke.

normally. Some patients are not aware of their memory problem, but their family and physician usually notice it, and it's obvious on memory testing. Mild cognitive impairment does not automatically mean a diagnosis of dementia or AD, but it's an extremely important warning sign.

Research studies have shown that in perhaps 40% of people with diagnosed mild cognitive impairment, the disorder will progress to AD within 3 years. People with such a diagnosis should remain under the care of a neurologist (a physician specializing in treatment of nervous system disorders).

32. What is normal-pressure hydrocephalus?

Normal-pressure hydrocephalus is another example of a dementing disease that can be reversed if it's detected early and is properly treated. Hydrocephalus means a condition in which a patient develops an excess of **cerebrospinal fluid**. The cerebrospinal fluid surrounds the brain, creating a sort of dynamic liquid cushion that protects the brain by shielding it from the hard bones of your skull. Your brain produces this fluid, and any excess is removed into your bloodstream. If something abruptly blocks the cerebrospinal fluid from being absorbed, it produces acute hydrocephalus with severe headache and increased pressure on the brain. If the mismatch between production and absorption of the cerebrospinal fluid is slight but evolves over time, your brain accommodates to a new condition that results in hydrocephalus (more fluid) but under normal or only slightly elevated pressure: the normal-pressure hydrocephalus.

Cerebrospinal fluid

fluid surrounding and cushioning the brain. It becomes altered in various brain diseases; therefore, investigation of cerebrospinal fluid may give a physician clues to diagnosis.

The symptoms of normal-pressure hydrocephalus include gait difficulties, urinary incontinence, and dementia. The gait difficulties include slowing of gait and decreasing length of strides with shuffling steps. This type of gait is called by neurologists a "magnetic gait," because such patients' feet appear to be constantly pulled toward the ground, as if by a magnet. Patients frequently report a feeling that they have to stop because they cannot walk any longer.

This becomes evident when, after being asked to walk during an examination, patients take shorter and shorter steps and eventually stop after several yards. Interestingly, if a physician holds them under an arm and walks alongside trying to pace their gait, such patients are capable of continuing to walk. These gait difficulties are usually the first symptoms of the disease, and after a time urinary incontinence starts.

In the type of urinary incontinence (discussed in Question 83) associated with normal-pressure hydrocephalus, patients are unable consciously to overcome the urge to urinate when their bladder is full and frequently are indifferent to wetting themselves. By the time urinary incontinence starts, the cognitive deficit is usually severe. The type of dementia associated with normal-pressure hydrocephalus equally involves memory, language, problem solving, and calculation. The first clue leading toward the correct diagnosis comes from nervous system examination and evaluation of the course of the disease; the second comes from imaging studies of the brain, which show increased spaces containing the cerebrospinal fluid.

Shunt

drainage device placed in the brain to remove excess cerebrospinal fluid and used to treat (among other disorders) normal-pressure hydrocephalus.

Cisternogram

study performed to investigate whether a patient with normal-pressure hydrocephalus would be a good candidate for a shunting procedure. During this test, a small amount of radioisotope is injected into the cerebrospinal fluid, and physicians using a special camera may determine signs of cerebrospinal fluid flow blockage.

Radioisotope

compound emitting radioactivity, therefore detectable by special camera. Radioisotopes are used for certain medical investigations (e.g., cysternogram) in evaluating normal-pressure hydrocephalus.

The treatment of normal-pressure hydrocephalus is surgical and involves inserting a small drain (a **shunt**) through which excess fluid can be removed from the brain. Usually, the fluid is drained into the abdominal cavity or the heart. Because the surgery is an invasive procedure with serious risks, a doctor has to be sure that placing a shunt device (discussed in Question 57) will likely produce a favorable result. To judge whether one would be a good candidate for the shunting procedure, a physician can perform a spinal tap (discussed in Question 44) and remove about 20 to 30 ml of cerebrospinal fluid, a lot like inserting a permanent drain. Immediately after removal of the cerebrospinal fluid, the patient would be asked to walk. The time and number of steps you made while walking a standardized distance would be recorded and compared to your performance before the spinal tap. The doctor might then perform a study called a **cisternogram** if the spinal tap produced a significant improvement. During the cisternogram, the doctor would inject a small amount of **radioisotope** into your cerebrospinal fluid and use a special camera that can see any signs of blockage of your cerebrospinal fluid flow.

The cisternogram takes 2 days to complete. Pictures are taken over several hours, 1 and 2 days after injection of the radioisotope. If the cisternogram results clearly picture normal-pressure hydrocephalus and the patient's gait showed significant improvement after a spinal tap, a shunting procedure probably would have a favorable outcome. If the shunting is successful, the gait difficulties improve, urinary incontinence disappears, and cognitive symptoms lessen.

The earlier the doctor performs a shunting procedure during the course of disease, the more likely a good outcome will occur. If a patient is in the stage of only mild gait difficulties with minor cognitive problems, shunting in normal-pressure hydrocephalus most likely would produce a very good result. However, if the workup is put off until a patient is bedridden and has severe dementia, your chances for improvement would be very poor.

33. What is Creutzfeldt-Jakob disease?

Creutzfeldt-Jakob disease is a rare condition occurring in one per million per year in the general population. It rapidly leads to dementia and death. In this disorder, a protein called "PrP," present in high amounts in nerve cells, undergoes specific rearrangement of its molecular structure. This renders the PrP indestructible, toxic, and capable of depositing in the brain, which leads to the death of neural cells. The disease can be spontaneous or inherited if one is born with a mutated form of this protein or as the result of infection when PrP in its abnormal form is passed from one person to another. Because destroying PrP is extremely difficult, accidental infection can be spread by contaminated surgical instruments previously used for brain surgery on a patient with Creutzfeldt-Jakob disease or by transplantation of a tissue part from such a patient. Such events (luckily very rare now) have occurred in the past when a patient was already infected with Creutzfeldt-Jakob disease but symptoms of the disease were not evident.

Recently, a number of people in Great Britain became ill with a new form of Creutzfeldt-Jakob disease after eating beef containing abnormal PrP from cows ill with "mad cow disease." An abnormal form of PrP protein also causes mad cow disease. Clinically, dementia

The earlier the doctor performs a shunting procedure during the course of disease, the more likely a good outcome will occur.

Risk Factors, Symptoms, and Diagnosis

related to the Creutzfeldt-Jakob disease has a much faster course than that of AD. On average, it takes 7 months from the onset of symptoms until death.

The symptoms of dementia in this disease are frequently seen as problems of balance, as seizures, and as jerky movements of the limbs. The disease does not spread through routine human-to-human contact; therefore, caring for patients who are sick with this disease does not pose an infectious hazard. Currently, no treatment for Creutzfeldt-Jakob disease exists.

34. What is apolipoprotein E? Should I be tested for the E isotype?

Apolipoprotein E is a protein that binds and transports cholesterol. Cholesterol makes up some 25% of all chemical substances building the brain and is vital for the proper functioning of nerve cells. Apolipoprotein E delivers cholesterol to nerve cells that need it. Research has also shown that apolipoprotein E can bind amyloid-β and effectively remove an excess from the brain. Therefore, apolipoprotein E has a protective function in preventing the brain from a buildup of amyloid-β. Apolipoprotein E exists in three forms (also called **isoforms** of apolipoprotein E): E2, E3, and E4. Differences in the chemical makeup between the three isoforms of apolipoprotein E are small but have a tremendous impact on AD.

Isoform

an alternate form of a protein showing minute differences in chemical composition. For example, apolipoprotein E may exist in three isoforms—E2, E3, and E4—in humans.

Apolipoprotein E isoforms are encoded by genes. Because each person has two copies of each gene encoding specific proteins, those with the following combinations of apolipoprotein genes are found: E2/E2; E3/E3; E4/E4; E2/E3; E2/E4; and E3/E4. Close to 60% of the general population have the

E3/E3 combination. Tests have shown that those people with one copy of the apolipoprotein E4 isoform (combinations E2/E4, E3/E4) have a four to five times greater chance for developing AD. People carrying two copies of apolipoprotein E4 (E4/E4) have an increased risk for sporadic AD about 17 times greater. Approximately 2% of the general population have the E4/E4 combination. Also, people with one or two copies of apolipoprotein E4 tend to develop AD symptoms earlier. This difference means a greater likelihood of developing dementia in the late sixties and early seventies for E4 carriers as opposed to an onset of AD in the late seventies and eighties for non–E4 carriers. Having one or two copies of the apolipoprotein E4 isoform certainly is a risk factor for the disease, but it does not automatically mean that E4 carriers will develop AD. AD is a sporadic disease, and the E4 isoform increases chances for its occurrence; however, some 50% of E4 carriers will never develop AD.

Why apolipoprotein E4 is a risk factor for AD is not fully understood. Experiments have shown that the E4 isoform is linked to impaired (reduced) removal of amyloid-β from the brain and promotes deposits of amyloid-β in plaques. In addition, recent evidence has shown that older apolipoprotein E4 carriers seem to have fewer connections between nerve cells, making the brain more vulnerable to AD damage. These properties of the apolipoprotein E4 isoform may shift the delicate balance between amyloid-β clearance versus amyloid-β deposits in older people, making it easier for the disease to develop.

As discussed, carriers of one copy of the apolipoprotein E4 gene have approximately a fourfold increased chance for developing sporadic AD, whereas carrying two copies of the apolipoprotein E4 gene increases the risk approximately 17-fold. A test for the apolipoprotein E type can be easily performed on blood and is commercially available from Athena Diagnostic for a cost of around $400. The usefulness of this test performed on healthy aged people or even on AD patients remains very questionable. You should be aware that fewer than 50% of E4 isoform carriers will develop AD and, conversely, that those who are not E4 carriers are not free from the possibility of developing AD. In other words, the presence of the apolipoprotein E4 gene is neither necessary nor sufficient for the diagnosis of AD.

Some cognitively normal persons who have heard about apolipoprotein E genotyping are asking for this test. Their doctors should consciously inform them about the interpretation of the test results and the fact that this test does not provide any certain answer. Although we do agree with our patients' wishes to analyze their apolipoprotein status, we also always make clear to them that finding that they have an apolipoprotein E4 genotype may elicit unnecessary stress and anxiety.

In summary, checking the apolipoprotein E genotype in patients with diagnosed AD does not have great clinical use. A negative analysis result does not exclude an AD diagnosis; although a positive result increases the possibility of AD somewhat, other diseases may also be at the cause (discussed in Question 28).

35. What is homocysteine?

Homocysteine is a molecule that is a normal metabolic breakdown product and is actively removed from the body. It can be toxic when present at elevated levels. Most people are able to maintain homocysteine

Homocysteine

product of normal body metabolism actively removed from the body. An elevated level of homocysteine is toxic.

below toxic levels. Unfortunately, in some people, homocyteine levels are elevated as a result of complex metabolic and dietary processes. Elevated homocysteine levels can damage blood vessels. At high levels, homocysteine can speed the rate of cholesterol deposits in vessel walls, which in turn may result in a stroke or heart attack. Recent evidence also links elevated homocysteine levels with an increased risk for AD. Elevated homocysteine levels in midlife are a strong risk factor for the beginning of AD symptoms 10 to 20 years later. In addition, in persons who have elevated homocysteine and already have symptoms of AD, the disease appears to progress faster. Although this finding has not yet become a part of guidelines published by any medical society, the authors strongly recommend checking the homocysteine levels in patients between the ages of 45 and 55 years on at least two separate occasions.

Doctors should also check homocysteine levels in people with diagnosed AD. This requires an easy blood test that can be performed (together with routine blood work for cholesterol) and administered by a primary-care physician. Measuring homocysteine levels is normal medical practice in people with an early episode (younger than 55 years) of stroke or myocardial infarction (discussed in Question 12). The treatment of an elevated homocysteine level is simple and safe even with a life-long duration. Usually, a combination of vitamins B_6 and B_{12} and folic acid taken once a day is prescribed. The impact of treatment on homocysteine levels can be easily shown by retesting the level 2 to 3 months after the start of treatment. Many over-the-counter preparations containing vitamins in the B group do not contain enough doses of vitamins B_6 and B_{12} and folic acid to lower homocysteine levels successfully. Therefore, a physician should manage people with an elevated level of homocysteine.

36. Can depression mimic AD symptoms?

Depression is a disease seen in depressed mood and motivation (will power or urge to act) and lack of energy and drive. Frequently, it's linked to fear, increased anxiety, and feelings of hopelessness. Sleep disturbances are frequent: nightmares or decreased amounts of sleep at night (or both), early awakening, and difficulties in falling back to sleep. Sexual drive is usually diminished. Depression in such persons usually limits attention and motivation; therefore, it also limits the amount of new information they can remember, as with patients with a memory disease, such as AD. The major difference is that in depression, patients have no internal drive to explore and memorize, whereas AD patients can't record information despite trying. Depression is related to deficiency of certain chemicals in nerve cells, called **neurotransmitters**, which those cells use to stimulate or inhibit each other. Unlike those with AD, depressed patients have no loss of nerve cells or buildup of abnormal proteins; therefore, use of proper chemicals in the form of a pill can reverse symptoms of depression. That's why depression is frequently called a "reversible dementia" in aged adults (discussed in Question 29). Depression is very common in older people, and each patient evaluated for dementia should be screened for symptoms of this disease. Depression is four times more likely to strike those older than 65 than younger individuals. It's found in 15% of adults older than 65. It coexists with AD in maybe 20% of patients. Moreover, depression

Neurotransmitter

chemical compound secreted at connections between nerve cells. There are either stimulatory or inhibitory neurotransmitters. By producing the former, a nerve cell may stimulate another nerve cell, whereas by producing the latter, a nerve cell may curb activity of another nerve cell.

affects up to 50% of AD caregivers (discussed in Question 90).

Many factors cause depression. For some people, the cause is an inborn risk for neurotransmitter imbalance. In such cases, the history of depression is lifelong, and such patients have had previous multiple episodes of worsening depression. In most other cases, depression can be a reaction to many things going on in life. Aged people who retire and engage in fewer social and professional activities are prone to develop depression. Typically, a doctor who evaluates a patient for a memory or other form of intellectual deficit and suspects that depression is the problem or is a contributing factor will start treatment with antidepressant medication or will refer the patient to be evaluated by a psychiatrist who specializes in the treatment of dementia. Many antidepressant medications are available on the market, and most patients tolerate them well and have only a few side effects. If treatment is successful, cognitive test scores should show improvements on behavioral tests within several weeks. Other treatments for depression include **psychotherapy**, which is based on conversations with a qualified therapist. The goal of psychotherapy is understanding the cause of depression in a particular individual and developing specific behavioral countermeasures, such as developing new interests or improving interpersonal skills.

Psychotherapy
therapy based on conversations between patient and therapist (frequently a psychiatrist) to understand the mechanism of psychological distress related to a mental illness (e.g., depression) and to create psychological countermeasures to combat it.

37. How is depression diagnosed?

The diagnosis of depression is made clinically, meaning that it is made on the basis of symptoms that a physician observes. No blood test or form of brain scan can back up the diagnosis of depression. Therefore, the physician's clinical experience is very important. The first step to diagnose depression in an elderly person being checked for cognitive damage is to realize that depression can be the cause of dementia or can lead to cognitive symptoms (discussed in Question 21 and 36). People with AD commonly exhibit symptoms of depression in the early stages of their disease, while they're still aware of the ongoing disease process. Because depression and dementia share common symptoms, the two are sometimes confused, with the result that depression often goes untreated in persons with AD. Many clinics and centers specializing in evaluation for dementia routinely perform on each patient a test called the **Hamilton depression scale**. It detects symptoms of depression and can show its magnitude. Unlike the Mini-Mental Scale Examination, the Hamilton depression scale has to be performed by a physician, nurse practitioner, or psychologist who is trained in asking the right questions and grading the responses. The examiner administers the Hamilton depression scale over 20 to 30 minutes, during that time asking the patient 20 questions to judge the most obvious symptoms of depression. These questions include information about depressed mood; feelings of guilt; having thoughts that life has no value; having thoughts about suicide; and about problems with sleep (falling asleep, waking up frequently, or waking up early in the morning and having difficulties in falling asleep again). Other parts of the evaluation for depression cover poor performance at work; withdrawal from activities; slowness; increased fear and anxiety; abdominal pain or diarrhea or different forms of pain; decreased sexual drive; and changes in weight. Feeling better in the evening than in the morning is typical for depression. A

Hamilton depression scale

clinical scale used to measure severity of depression.

physician should treat with antidepressants such patients who demonstrate symptoms of depression. Cognitive tests repeated after several weeks can demonstrate the impact of depression on mental performance. A correct diagnosis and a proper antidepressant should improve memory scores on repeated testing.

38. What should I expect after a diagnosis of AD?

Accepting the diagnosis of a disease is always difficult, especially if your diagnosis is that of a progressing, currently incurable illness. Centers and clinics dedicated to the diagnosis and management of AD give patients many opportunities to learn about the disease (discussed in Questions 1, 7, 8, and 100) and to ask questions not only of physicians but of nurses and social workers. Patients and their caregivers have to understand that AD is not a normal part of aging but a degenerative disease of the brain that affect memory, thinking, and behavior; this impairment has a progressive (worsening) character. Although there is no cure for the disease, some of its symptoms can be treated by medications and behavioral approaches. These behavioral approaches are aimed at reducing anxiety and agitation, which are associated with progression of AD (discussed in Questions 69 and 70).

Doctors should discuss with you how the disease may progress and offer a specific plan for future care and follow-up. Social workers will provide you with written educational materials and a list of available community resources, including the Alzheimer's Disease Association (discussed in Question 94). They always allow sufficient time to answer questions from affected individuals and their families. They may need to schedule a follow-up meeting with you to continue discussions.

39. What doctor should I see for help? How often?

Geriatrician

internist specializing in medical problems of elderly individuals.

Three medical specialties can be involved in evaluating and caring for patients with AD: a **geriatrician** (a specialist in general medical problems of the elderly), a neurologist (a specialist in the nervous system), and a geriatric psychiatrist (a specialist in mental diseases of the elderly). Most patients have a primary care physician who is responsible for maintaining their general health and detecting early such conditions as elevated blood pressure, diabetes, and elevated cholesterol. Frequently, after detecting a problem on a routine medial examination or when prompted by a concerned family member, primary care physicians will refer patients to a neurologist who will weigh their memory problems. You should see your primary care physician at least once a year for a check-up. If you don't see your primary care physician on a regular basis or have concerns about your memory (discussed in Questions 17 and 18), you can seek neurological advice on your own. For making the diagnosis of AD and excluding other diseases that can be similar to AD, a neurologist is typically best suited.

You should see your primary care physician at least once a year for a check-up.

There are many ways for you to find an appropriate specialist. You can ask your primary-care physician or explore the Web site of the nearest comprehensive medical center (discussed in the Appendix). Each large medical center has a referral guide available by phone or through a medical center Web page. *U.S. News & World Report* yearly publishes a list of the top 50 medical centers in each specialty. By searching at *http://www.usnews.com/usnews/nycu/health/hosptl/rankings/specihqneur.htm*, you can find the ranking of various departments of neurology in a medical center near you. An additional important resource is the local Alzheimer's Disease Association chapter. The Alzheimer's Disease Web site is located at *http://www. alz.org* (800-272-3900).

Also, 29 Alzheimer's disease research centers are located throughout the United States, all working with the National Institute of Aging. These centers are excellent for the diagnosis and treatment of AD. A list of these centers is available at *http://www. alzheimers.org/adcdir.htm*.

How often patients see a physician depends on their diagnosis. If an AD diagnosis is made, they should remain under the care of a neurologist who will administer cholinesterase inhibitors (discussed in Questions 51–54), monitor response to treatment, assess progression of the disease, and examine patients for associated conditions (e.g., behavioral problems). Treatment with cholinesterase inhibitors (discussed in Question 51) requires seeing a neurologist every 3 to 6 months. If such patients have both AD and vascular dementia (see Question 30) or show behavioral symptoms that require treatment with **neuroleptics**, their doctor may have to schedule more frequent visits. Sometimes, behavioral symptoms may require treatment by geriatric psychiatrists who specialize in treating agitation and depression associated with dementia. Depending on how severe their problems are, affected patients

Neuroleptics

class of medications used to treat hallucinations, delusions, and agitation in AD patients.

should see their primary-care physician every 6 to 12 months or even more frequently. A primary-care physician is either an internist or a geriatrician (an internist specializing in treating older adults). A primary-care physician will monitor blood pressure, cholesterol, and glucose (blood sugar) levels to make sure that a patient is not developing hypertension (see Question 19), heart disease, or diabetes. If any of these may be a problem, the doctor will begin appropriate treatment, will ensure that vaccinations against flu and pneumonia are up to date, and will perform cancer screens, as advancing age increases the risk of various types of cancer.

40. If I'm scheduled to see a neurologist, what should I expect?

If you go to a neurologist (specialist in the nervous system) with a chief complaint of memory problems, you can be placed in any of three groups: (1) you don't have dementia but are concerned about age-related memory deficiency; (2) you have AD or another treatable or nontreatable form of dementia (discussed in Questions 28 and 29); or (3) you have memory problems resulting from depression or anxiety. Your neurologist would have to decide in which of these groups you fit and, if your symptoms signal dementia, should be able to diagnose its type.

As discussed, no test can clearly make or rule out a diagnosis of AD, and certain conditions may overlap with early AD and depression. Therefore, a process of evaluation performed by a neurologist is detailed and complete. A visit to a neurologist for memory problems would typically involve recording a careful history of the nature of problems and their duration. If you had any written record of previous treatments, laboratory results, or imaging results, you should bring them with you to the appointment. Your neurologist would also ask about other diseases and about medications you're taking, as well as your occupation and any family history of dementing illnesses.

You would be tested for memory and other intellectual functions using short tests (including the Mini-Mental Status Examination). Testing for depression is routinely performed as well. Your doctor would measure your heart rate, temperature, and blood pressure; perform a neurological examination to check the function of your nerves, gait, and balance; and then order a number of additional tests (discussed in Question 45).

41. What is the reason for the blood tests the doctor ordered?

A neurologist routinely recommends some blood work as part of the workup (diagnosis process) for a memory problem. The number of tests would depend on when the most recent complete blood tests were performed by a primary-care physician and whether these results are available. Evaluations include a general blood count, liver function, electrolytes, glucose (blood sugar), and cholesterol as well as tests more specific for dementia (e.g., thyroid hormones, levels of vitamin B_{12} and its associated **metabolite** methylmalonic acid), and homocysteine (discussed in Question 35). A low level of thyroid hormones or vitamin B_{12} is a reversible cause of dementia (discussed in Question 29). Rarely, either of these problems alone is responsible for symptoms of dementia. More frequently, a partial lack, which is more frequent in the aged population, may coexist with AD and add to the level of cognitive

Metabolite

product of chemical reaction taking place in the body.

impairment. These conditions are treatable and, in most cases, reversible. Many doctors would also send out a test for syphilis. That's because (in rare cases) syphilis infection may remain unrecognized for long periods and, if not treated correctly, may cause dementia 10 to 30 years after the initial infection. Because of the importance of vascular dementia (discussed in Question 30) and the impact of high cholesterol, diabetes, and homocysteine levels on the onset and course of AD, a doctor would also focus on checking blood glucose, cholesterol, and homocysteine levels.

42. Why do I need a brain scan?

Your physician can order four types of brain scans: computed tomography (CT) scan, magnetic resonance imaging (MRI), single-photon emission computed tomography (SPECT), and positron emission tomography (PET) scan. The first two—CT and MRI— show the *structure* of your brain; SPECT and PET provide insights into the *activity* of particular areas of your brain. MRI rather than CT is preferred in evaluating dementia because the picture of your brain that it provides is of unmatched resolution and accuracy.

Doctors can obtain several different types of data from MRI images. This method can show us whether you've undergone any strokes in the past and can reveal the extent of small-vessel disease (discussed in Question 30). In this way, doctors can decide whether this is a vascular type of dementia. MRI can also show, with high resolution, atrophy (wasting) of the hippocampus, an area of your brain that's severely affected by AD. The MRI finding of decreased volume in the hippocampus can be helpful in predicting whether your mild cognitive impairment is likely to progress to AD.

Enlarged ventricles may suggest normal-pressure hydrocephalus. Although brain tumors may produce dementia, this occurs extremely rarely. Moreover, brain tumors tend to show up with such other symptoms as limb weakness and vision loss rather than pure memory problems. A neurologist (a specialist in nervous system diseases) finding evidence of an old stroke may order other tests to investigate the condition of your heart and large arteries, where disease could have triggered the stroke. If the MRI clearly shows normal-pressure hydrocepahalus (discussed in Question 32), your doctor would perform further testing.

People with **pacemakers, automatic implanted cardiodefibrillators**, and certain metal implants cannot have MRI because the study is performed in a powerful magnetic field. Apart from these exemptions, no evidence proves that short-term exposure to high magnetic fields can be harmful. For persons who suffer from claustrophobia, MRI may be difficult because it requires entering a confined space. Mild sedation, an open MRI, or CT are alternatives for these patients.

SPECT and PET are highly specialized tests that can document the metabolism of brain areas. SPECT shows the rate of your metabolism (energy usage) by measuring blood flow supply; PET directly measures the body's use of glucose (blood sugar) by nerve cells. In both tests, a doctor injects a small amount of **radioisotope** into the bloodstream, and special sensors detect the level of **radioactivity**. The amount of radioactivity used during these tests is very small. A

Pacemaker

device implanted in certain patients with heart problems for controlling heart rate. Installing a pacemaker prohibits the use of magnetic resonance imaging.

Automatic implanted cardiac defibrillator

device implanted into a patient's chest that is able to detect life-threatening abnormalities of cardiac rhythm and automatically deliver small electric shocks to bring heart rhythm back to normal.

Radio-isotope

compound emitting radioactivity that is detectable by a special camera.

computer translates information from many sensors into brain maps to show the local level of metabolism. Brain areas with high nerve cell loss due to neurodegenerative disease usually show a reduction in both blood flow (seen on SPECT) and glucose use (seen on PET). An MRI finding of atrophy in the hippocampus and a PET finding of hypometabolism strongly suggest a diagnosis of AD. These tests, however, have a limited sensitivity in the early stages of the disease.

43. What's the purpose of psychological testing?

Neurologists may recommend psychological testing for you.

Neurologists may recommend psychological testing for you. Its purpose is to measure your performance in memory and other aspects of cognition. Persons trained in clinical psychology perform such tests, and the testing usually lasts 2 to 3 hours. They analyze memory by having patients perform a variety of tasks, including listening to and repeating short stories and learning pairs of words, objects, or colors and objects. They weigh language function by having patients name a number of words in a limited period, describe the meaning of less commonly used words, and write sentences. They administer different graphic tasks to judge ability to process images. They use simple mathematical tasks to check ability to calculate and solve problems. They run these tests from the easiest to the most difficult and grade them accordingly.

Testing may answer questions about the severity of cognitive deficit and suggest the type of dementia the doctors suspect. Testing also excludes mild cognitive impairment when there's a question between early dementia and normal aging (discussed in Question 7).

The pattern of damage is different in AD, vascular dementia, and depression. Evident in depression is that a patient doesn't put enough effort into memorizing and solving tasks. Depression produces obvious difficulties with focusing and concentration. Conversely, in AD, a patient tries hard to solve a problem and memorize data but performs poorly. We recommend performing extended behavioral testing during the first session. If depression is likely, the scores on behavioral testing should improve under treatment with antidepressants. If testing confirms AD or another degenerative illness, a psychologist should periodically repeat testing in a simplified form to judge the progression of the disease and any response to treatment. One of the most frequently used simple tests for cognitive evaluation and follow-up is the Mini-Mental State Examination Test. This test performed by a trained professional takes approximately 10 minutes and weighs many cognitive areas. The format of this test is given below.

Orientation (5 points each)

( ) Ask patient, "what is the (year) (season) (day) (date) (month)?"

( ) Ask patient, "where are we (state) (county) (town) (hospital) (floor)?"

Registration (3 points)

( ) Ask patient to name three unrelated objects. Allow 1 second to say each. Then ask the patient to repeat all three after you have said them. Give one point for each correct answer. Repeat them until he or she learns all three.

(continues)

Attention

( ) Ask patient to count backward from 100 by sevens. Give one point for each correct answer. Stop after five answers. Or, spell the word *world* backwards. *Remember: This task is to evaluate attention span, not calculation. Attention span is the ability to carry out the task continuously. If the patient during serial subtractions gives following answers 93, 86, 78 (instead of 79), 71, and 64, you can give five points. You should give two points if patient stops on 86 and requires a cue to continue counting.*

Recall

( ) Ask patient to recall the three objects previously stated. Give one point for each correct answer. *You can see the difference between the process of registration, which is a test for working memory, and recall, which tests ability to consolidate (i.e., practically making new memories).*

Language

( ) Show patient a wrist watch; ask patient what it is. Repeat for a pencil. (2 points)

( ) Ask patient to repeat the following: "No ifs, ands, or buts." (1 point)

( ) Ask patient to follow a three-stage command: "Take a paper in your right hand, fold it in half, and put it on the floor." (3 points)

( ) Ask patient to read and obey the following sentence written on a piece of paper: "Close your eyes." (1 point)

( ) Ask patient to write a sentence. (1 point)

(continues)

Visual skills

( ) Ask patient to copy a design. (1 point)

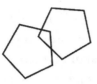

Total number of points _____

The maximal number of points on the Mini-Mental State Examination is 30. A range of between 26 and 30 is found in cognitively normal subjects. This wide range depends on intelligence and level of education. The Mini-Mental State Examination has to be applied with common sense. A score of 26 may mean cognitive impairment in somebody with a university degree, whereas this same score in somebody who finished education at the primary school level can be normal. Certainly, in everybody a score below 25 is a sure sign of mild to moderate cognitive impairment, whereas a score of 17 and below means severe cognitive impairment.

44. What information can a spinal tap provide?

The spinal tap (also called lumbar puncture) is a procedure performed to obtain a sample of your cerebrospinal fluid. Because cerebrospinal fluid surrounds your brain, its chemical makeup faithfully reflects many conditions taking place in your brain. Doctors remove a small sample of fluid through a long thin needle introduced into your lower back area. For the spinal tap, you'd either lie on one side or sit bent forward. The site where the needle is inserted is numbed with a local anesthetic, and the skin is cleaned with an antiseptic agent. After the spinal tap, you'd have to lie flat for a minimum of 30 minutes.

Rare complications of this procedure include headache (prevented by lying flat), infection, and sciatica.

In AD, the level of amyloid-β in cerebrospinal fluid decreases, and the level of tau protein (involved in formation of neurofibrillary tangles; discussed in Question 9) increases. These changes are very typical for AD. In contrast, in frontotemporal dementia, the amyloid-β level is unchanged, and only the tau protein level is increased. In vascular dementia (discussed in Question 30), the levels of both proteins are normal.

Analysis of amyloid-β and tau levels in the cerebrospinal fluid is commercially available. Although this test seems to produce fairly accurate results, its sensitivity is limited, especially in the stage of mild cognitive impairment. Hence, the values become abnormal when the clinical picture of the AD type of dementia becomes fairly clear. Therefore, this test adds only a little to the information obtained from clinical examination, MRI, and psychological testing. Although possible complications are few, they still exist. The spinal tap is usually not recommended unless your doctor suspects that dementia may be related to or complicated by infection, inflammation, or spreading tumor. In such instances, doctors perform the spinal tap to exclude the aforementioned conditions while at the same time possibly sending a sample to the laboratory for measuring amyloid-β and tau levels to confirm an AD diagnosis.

45. When should genetic testing be performed?

Genetic testing is not a part of the routine workup (diagnosis process) for AD. In some 95% of AD cases, the disease occurs by chance (in other words, is sporadic) and isn't related to a specific gene abnormality. Although apolipoprotein E isoform testing is available, the presence of an apolipoprotein E4 isoform is neither necessary nor enough for the diagnosis of sporadic AD. Genetic testing should be performed only in rare situations in which AD patients demonstrate an onset of dementia symptoms before the age of 65. These patients frequently have many close relatives affected by AD, which raises another red flag suggesting the possibility of a genetic defect running in the entire family.

In some 95% of AD cases, the disease occurs by chance and isn't related to a specific gene abnormality.

Mutations (inherited genetic defects) of one of three genes—presenilin 1, presenilin 2, and the amyloid precursor protein (discussed in Question 11)—can be involved in early-onset AD. Of these three genes, presenilin 1 mutations are the most common cause for early-onset AD. Testing for presenilin 1 mutations is performed from a blood sample and is commercially available. Most AD experts recommend testing for genetic mutations for all those who develop AD before the age of 65. Most of these genetic mutations are inherited in an **autosomal dominant** fashion, meaning that almost all people who inherit a presenilin 1 mutation will eventually develop AD if they live long enough. Therefore, siblings or children of an AD patient who show no symptoms and whose genetic testing showed presenilin 1 mutation can also be offered genetic testing. Before a doctor orders a test, if patients are healthy, they should go through genetic counseling so that they understand both the benefits and the consequences of this type of testing. A negative result on the test means that they won't develop early-onset AD, but their chance for developing sporadic AD is similar to that for the general population. If the test results comes back positive, however, they'd

Autosomal dominant

the way in which genetic diseases are inherited. Genes usually exist in pairs, called alleles. In autosomal dominant genetic diseases, passing only one mutated allele (gene copy) is sufficient to produce disease in the next generation. In contrast, autosomal recessive diseases occur only if two alleles (gene copies) are affected.

have to live knowing that they'll eventually get sick with an irreversible illness. Therefore, many people placed in such a situation decide not to undergo genetic testing.

In perhaps 50% of familial, early-onset AD cases, no mutations can be detected in presenilin 1, presenilin 2, or the amyloid precursor protein genes. These cases are related to mutations in genes yet to be discovered. Currently, this is an area of intense research.

PART THREE

Treatment

Can I prevent AD?

What are the goals of AD treatment?

What is the vaccine for AD?

More ...

RISK REDUCTION AND PREVENTION

46. Can taking vitamins reduce the risk of AD? If so, what vitamins should I take?

Many years of research have shown that in generally healthy persons, diet alone can readily meet nutritional needs. Therefore, guidelines from many professional societies or governmental panels recommend attempting to obtain vitamins and minerals from food sources rather than from supplements. Unfortunately, many aging people experience some age-related changes in food absorption and metabolism that may lead to partial lack of certain vitamins. Also, several large medical trials have demonstrated the benefits of taking some vitamins for reducing the chance of developing some age-related diseases. The American Dietetic Association and the U.S. Dietary Guidelines suggest that some people may need vitamin or mineral supplements, in addition to a good diet, to ensure that they meet their optimal nutritional needs.

As discussed in Question 35, vitamins B_6, B_{12}, and folic acid reduce homocysteine levels and prevent vascular diseases. In addition, a higher intake of folic acid is thought to lower your risk for developing colon and breast cancers. In older people, owing to decreased absorption, the level of vitamin B_{12} is frequently low. A low level of vitamin B_{12} is linked to an increased occurrence of vascular diseases, certain forms of cancer, and dementia. Therefore, the level of this vitamin is particularly interesting for a neurologist evaluating you for memory problems. Vitamins from the B group are especially plentiful in meat, cereal, and legumes. Also, many elderly people have a lack of vitamin D, a lack that according to many studies can increase your risk of fractures. Vitamins E and C have **antioxidant** properties, which means these vitamins are able to neutralize free radicals (toxic by-products of many metabolic reactions in your body). One theory about why aging occurs points to free radicals as damaging cells and their parts. Supplementing your diet with 400 UI of vitamin E for 2 years has been shown to reduce significantly your risk for heart attacks and prostate cancer. Vitamin C may be beneficial also in combating heart disease and certain types of cancer. Both vitamins C and E have been found to prevent AD and to slow its course. Large clinical studies haven't demonstrated a significant benefit of vitamins C and E in AD, but many physicians prescribe vitamin E in those with clinically diagnosed AD. Vitamin E intake of up to 1,000 IU daily is considered safe.

Antioxidant
compound capable of neutralizing free radicals. (See free radicals) Vitamin E is an example.

Treatment

The practice of taking daily multivitamin preparations makes sense for aged adults taking into account the greater likelihood of benefit than harm and considering their low cost. Many preparations are available. You should keep in mind that the U.S. Food and Drug Administration (FDA) regulates production and distribution of dietary supplements only to a limited degree; therefore, in many situations, over-the-counter preparations lack quality control. We usually recommend that you select complex vitamin supplements from a reputable brand of your choice. We also evaluate our patients for possible age-related vitamin deficiencies; if they're discovered, we treat them with pharmacy-obtained vitamin formulas.

47. Should I perform memory exercises?

Like many other systems in your body, your brain—especially its memory function—possesses some flexibility, which you can increase by stimulation and exercise. As discussed in Question 15, the rate of AD is lower among people with higher education. By this line of thinking, you may ask whether performing memory exercises or being involved in intellectually stimulating activities can reduce your odds for developing AD. Indeed, results of several research studies suggest that frequent participation in activities that stimulate your mind is associated with reducing your risk of AD twofold. In one such study, a group consisting of more than 2,800 older adults participated in an experiment to assess the value of the following cognitive skills that help in the activities of daily living: training of memory, speed of processing, and reasoning. The participants were evaluated before the training began, after the training was completed, and then 1 and 2 years later. A significant improvement in cognitive skills was found in those participants as compared to others in a group that did not receive training. The improvements continued to persist even 2 years after training.

It's extremely important to remain involved in such stimulating activities as you get older. The range of these activities may involve daily reading, developing new hobbies, or studying new subjects. Some AD centers offer so-called memory exercises performed in either group or individual sessions under the guidance of a psychologist and directed at improving your functions of learning and memory. Participants in these sessions are recruited from either older adults with complaints about subjective memory problems or patients in the early stages of AD. Performing such activities regularly has some beneficial impact on the symptoms of early AD and mild cognitive impairment (discussed in Question 31).

48. Does hormone replacement therapy help to prevent AD?

Researchers have established that receptors for **estrogens** (female sexual hormones) and for **testosterone** (male sexual hormone) are present on nerve cells, especially those in your hippocampus. These hormones seem to be directly involved in the well-being of your brain's nerve cells. Therefore, it was not a surprise that animals with low sexual hormone levels show limited performance on behavioral memory testing. Levels of sexual hormones naturally decline with aging. In women, these changes have a more abrupt character linked to the menopause, whereas in men production of testosterone decreases slowly over time.

Some physicians started to question the relationship between declining levels of sexual hormones and the chance for developing AD and whether hormone replacement therapy could be helpful. Over the last 50 years, hormone replacement therapy for the treatment of the symptoms of menopause has created a great deal of controversy. Such therapy relieves most of the subjective complaints (hot flashes, problems with concentration, mood swings) and improves general well-being. This therapy also prevents **osteoporosis**, reducing your chances of bone fracture.

On the basis of small-scale studies, physicians used to believe that hormone replacement therapy reduces the chances for heart attacks. They found a lower rate of

Estrogen
female sexual hormone.

Testosterone
male sexual hormone.

Osteoporosis
weakening of bones usually associated with aging and brought on by hormonal changes taking place during menopause in women.

AD in those women who were taking hormone preparations for 10 years or more, but not in those taking hormones for less than 10 years. Surprisingly, in July of 2002, a very large, multicenter trial examining the risks and benefits of combined estrogen and progestin in healthy menopausal women was stopped early. The study found an increased risk of invasive breast cancer and modest increases in the rate of heart attacks, strokes, and **pulmonary embolism**. The study compared participants taking estrogen plus progestin to women taking placebo pills. There were noteworthy benefits of hormone replacement therapy, including fewer cases of hip fractures and colon cancer, but on balance the harm was greater than the benefit. The study also did not confirm the benefit of hormone replacement therapy on the incidence of AD. More research is needed before definitive recommendations can be made to female patients, especially when considering these recent studies linking a number of health risks with the hormone replacement therapy use.

Pulmonary embolism

serious medical condition caused by closing off a lung artery by an embolus. Symptoms include chest pain and breathing difficulties.

No hormone replacement therapy is currently recommended for men. It appears, however, that higher levels of free testosterone may protect against specific types of memory decline in elderly men. Researchers need to understand much more about how testosterone levels affect the aging brain and body before doctors begin recommending treatment. It's not known whether hormone replacement therapy for men, if such would ever be introduced, would have a similar negative impact on their rate of heart disease and cancer, as does hormone replacement therapy for women. Experience gathered from previous clinical trials suggests caution.

Researchers need to understand much more about how testosterone levels affect the aging brain and body before doctors begin recommending treatment.

49. Can taking anti-inflammatory drugs prevent AD?

Epidemiological studies showed there is a lower rate of AD among people taking anti-inflammatory drugs (ibuprofen, diclofenac, or naproxyn) for non-AD-related conditions. Those results gave rise to the notion that anti-inflammatory drugs prevent AD. These disorders for which anti-inflammatory drugs are commonly prescribed included various forms of arthritis involving hands, hips, knees, and spine, and different musculoskeletal pain syndromes. Both amyloid-β plaques and neurofibrillary tangles (discussed in Questions 5, 12, 14, and 30) in the brain of AD patients cause local inflammation that can harm nerve cells. Following this line of thinking, large clinical trials have investigated whether different classes of anti-inflammatory agents may slow down and possibly stop the development of AD. Unfortunately, no trial using the aforementioned older anti-inflammatory agents or even newer drugs (such as Celebrex) has shown a significant impact on AD progress so far. Several trials with other anti-inflammatory drugs are under way.

People who have been taking anti-inflammatory agents steadily for other medical problems may expect a significant decrease in their chance of developing AD if they've taken such drugs for 2 or more years. Such prolonged treatment is connected to an increased risk of major side effects, including massive digestive system bleeding. Therefore, we currently cannot recommend this form of prevention.

Treatment

MEDICATIONS FOR AD PATIENTS

50. What are the goals of AD treatment?

AD is a progressive process leading to the buildup of amyloid-β deposits and neurofibrillary tangles (discussed in Question 9). This buildup results in the death of nerve cells and at the same time in destruction of connections between nerve cells that are still alive. The ideal treatment option would arrest the process of built-up toxic proteins, preventing death in neurons and interruption of connections. Despite extensive research, this kind of treatment is still unavailable. Several groups of drugs helpful to AD patients are available, and their use is the current standard of care for AD patients. One large group of drugs improves the ability of neurons to communicate between themselves. This group includes the cholinesterase inhibitors and Memantine (discussed in the following questions). Although they do not stop the disease process, these drugs modestly improve cognitive performance and slow down progression of disease symptoms. Other groups of drugs designed to slow down the rate of AD are those used to eliminate **free radicals**, such as vitamin E and selegiline (discussed in Question 57).

Many other medications also are useful in the treatment of behavior problems arising from AD. These symptoms may vary in individuals and in the stage of the disease process. Various antidepressants can easily help with symptoms of depression, which can be linked to both early and moderately advanced AD. These drugs are usually well tolerated. As the disease progresses, outbursts of agitation (discussed in Question 69) and episodes of psychotic behavior—which may include paranoid thoughts, delusions, or halluci-

Free radicals

toxic metabolites of various chemical reactions taking place in the body. Inability to neutralize free radicals successfully is considered a reason for nerve death in certain neurodegenerative diseases (e.g., Parkinson's disease and, to a lesser extent, AD).

nations (discussed in Questions 72 and 73)—can become more frequent. They may be dangerous to AD patients and put stress on family and relationship ties. Uncontrolled agitation and psychotic episodes are some of the most frequent causes of admission to nursing facilities. However, antipsychotic medications can control and even prevent these symptoms.

The overall goal of all these treatment methods is to maintain the remaining cognitive ability at the highest level possible and to control behavioral symptoms. This allows patients to function in the home environment for as long as possible.

51. What are cholinesterase inhibitors?

Cholinesterase inhibitors are drugs that enter your brain and block an enzyme called "cholinesterase." The cholinesterase enzyme breaks down the **acetylcholine**, a substance that's produced by nerve cells and is absolutely vital for a functioning memory system. In AD patients, the level of acetylcholine is much lower than that in normal people. Thus, by blocking the cholinesterase, these inhibitors increase the amount of acetylcholine in the brain. In this way, these drugs lessen symptoms of dementia and slow down the clinical (but not biological) progression of AD. In other words, as death of nerve cells causes the symptoms of AD, cholinesterase inhibitors increase the amount of acetylcholine in those nerve cells that are still functioning, allowing them at least to make up partially for the loss. In this way, cholinesterase inhibitors lessen clinical symptoms of AD but do not stop the disease process.

Acetylcholine
an activating neuro-transmitter indispensable for the brain's cognitive process.

These drugs may also to a lesser degree control symptoms of agitation (discussed in Question 69). Four cholinesterase inhibitors are approved by the U.S.

Treatment

Food and Drug Administration (FDA): Cognex (tacrine), Aricept (donezepil), Exelon (rivastigmine), and Reminyl (galantamine). Cognex was the first drug from this class approved for clinical use, whereas Reminyl is the most recently introduced on the market. Besides inhibiting cholinesterase, Reminyl can act directly on acetylcholine receptors to increase their response to acetylcholine. All the cholinesterase inhibitors are available only in the form of tablets taken once or twice a day.

52. When should cholinesterase inhibitors be started?

Researchers showed the positive effect of cholinesterase inhibitors on cognitive (thinking) ability in patients with mild to moderately advanced AD; their scores on the Mini-Mental State Examination Test ranged from 10 to 26 points. Until recently, no reliable information covered the effect of these drugs on mild cognitive impairment. Recently published data suggest that taking cholinesterase inhibitors improves memory scores in people in this early stage. It's a passing stage between normal aging and AD (when patients experience only memory problems), whereas other intellectual functions remain fully intact. Because mild cognitive impairment converts to AD each year in some 15% of patients, some clinical researchers are optimistic that starting cholinesterase inhibitors early may delay AD onset. Therefore, many doctors are willing to prescribe cholinesterase inhibitors in very early stages of the disease, and these drugs are currently the standard of care for AD patients until they reach the advanced stages. In addition to delaying progression of

AD, cholinesterase inhibitors have been shown to work in improving cognitive performance and behavior in patients with vascular dementia (discussed in Question 30) and in patients with Lewy-body dementia (discussed in Question 28).

Doses of all cholinesterase inhibitors must be increased slowly, and preferred treatment is to start it at bedtime. This is done to avoid digestive system upset (such as nausea or vomiting). Aricept should be started at the dose of 5 mg at bedtime. This dose should be continued for 6 weeks and then advanced to 10 mg once a day at bedtime. Exelon should be started at the dose of 1.5 mg at bedtime for 2 weeks and then increased to 1.5 mg twice a day. Later dose increases should occur after each 2-week period, first to 3 mg twice a day, then to 4.5 mg twice a day, and finally to 6 mg twice a day. Treatment with Reminyl is begun with 4 mg at bedtime for 4 weeks; then the dose is increased to 4 mg twice a day. After another 4 weeks, the dose is doubled to 8 mg twice daily; then, if the patient tolerates it well, it may be raised after another 4 weeks to 12 mg twice a day, to a total daily dose of 24 mg. Because starting therapy with Exelon and Reminyl may appear overwhelming, owing to their complicated schedules and dosage increases, to avoid confusion companies producing these drugs offer so-called starting kits with different color-coded tablets containing increasing amounts of the drug and exact instructions. All cholinesterase inhibitors should be given with food. About 3 months after treatment begins, patients should undergo a follow-up neuropsychological testing (discussed in Question 43) to weigh the effect of treatment. Treatment with cholinesterase inhibitors should continue throughout the course of disease. It can be stopped in the end stages of AD, when these drugs no longer have an effect.

53. Are cholinesterase inhibitors safe?

Except for tacrine, cholinesterase inhibitors have a very good safety record and limited side effects and do not interact with most other drugs. What is also critical is that patients do not need to have periodic blood tests while on this therapy. This is extremely important because patients remain on cholinesterase inhibitors for many years. Tacrine is an exception because it's linked with possible liver damage. Currently, this drug is not prescribed often.

Anorexia
severe and prolonged lack of appetite leading to significant loss of weight and malnutrition. This condition can be life-threatening.

Once therapy with cholinesterase inhibitors begins, both patients and caregivers have to watch for the following unpleasant side effects: nausea, vomiting, diarrhea, **anorexia**, weight loss, dizziness, insomnia (sleeplessness), and urinary incontinence (loss of bladder control). Digestive system upset is the most frequent reason to stop therapy. The possibility of these not-very-serious but certainly unpleasant side effects can be reduced and avoided by increasing the dose slowly and giving drugs at night and with food. This is very important because experiencing these unpleasant (but not dangerous) symptoms can permanently discourage patients from taking these valuable drugs. A doctor also can use certain other means if AD patients develop unpleasant symptoms in their digestive system. For example, the drug dose can be increased much more slowly, taking smaller steps.

Some patients also respond well to switching from one drug to another. If nausea and vomiting are major problems, doctors can give patients **antiemetic medications**. These simple measures frequently work and could help many patients to continue therapy with cholinesterase inhibitors.

Only a few conditions would prevent the use of cholinesterase inhibitors: active peptic ulcer disease, unstable asthma or **chronic obstructive pulmonary disease,** and heart disease. Increased caution is recommended when these drugs are used with certain heart medications, such as digoxin or beta-blockers, or if a patient has a history of blackout or seizures. Patients also should stop using cholinesterase inhibitors for surgery because they might interfere with anesthesia. The drug should be stopped about 2 weeks prior to surgery and slowly resumed after recovery.

54. Is any cholinesterase inhibitor better than others?

Of the four cholinesterase inhibitors approved by the U.S. Food and Drug Administration (FDA), three are frequently prescribed: Aricept (donezepil), Exelon (rivastigmine), and Reminyl (galantamine). Cognex (tacrine) is available but, because of the remote possibility of producing liver damage requiring frequent liver function tests to monitor that organ, it's not often used. The other three cholinesterase inhibitors have a much more limited range of side effects and fewer cautions that would keep patients from using them. In clinical trials, Aricept, Exelon, and Reminyl showed a roughly similar degree of benefit. AD patients placed on one of these cholinesterase inhibitors showed modest improvement when tested using special research dementia scales, although their disease continued to

Antiemetic
medication given to stop or prevent nausea and vomiting.

Chronic obstructive pulmonary disease
prolonged bronchitis resulting from many years of smoking or exposure to toxic fumes. Symptoms include shortness of breath, gasping, and decreased exercise tolerance.

Treatment

progress. The disease in untreated patients in these trials had a much faster downhill course. On average, the use of these drugs extends an AD patient's level of function by about 6 months to 1 year.

Experience gained in clinical trials showed a relationship between the use of cholinesterase inhibitors and clinical effects. A dose of Aricept (5 mg/day) brought about improvement, and increasing the dose to 10 mg/day might produce a better effect. Exelon had no effect at a dose below 4 mg/day but was successful at 6 mg/day and 12 mg/day. Reminyl showed an effect at a dose of 8 mg/day, with a better effect at 12 mg/day and 24 mg/day. All these drugs have been investigated separately. Clinical trials are being organized to compare them head-to-head but, until results are published, no one can clearly state whether one drug is distinctly better than another. Clinical experience suggests that all have similar benefits at the optimal dose. Choice of a particular drug depends on the treating physician's decision as to how to tailor the drug to the range of a patient's symptoms. For example, Exelon has a mild tranquilizing effect and may be a better choice for those patients for whom agitation (discussed in Questions 69 and 70) is a significant problem.

Often, caregivers report that they do not see a significant improvement after a cholinesterase inhibitor has been started.

Often, caregivers report that they do not see a significant improvement after a cholinesterase inhibitor has been started. One must understand that the effect of these drugs is typically to slow down the progression of symptoms, something that may take some time to be noticeable. Cholinesterase inhibitors require several weeks until the desired dose is achieved. We recommend that the dose be increased slowly and gradually to avoid stomach upset. Treatment with cholinesterase inhibitors is part of the standard medical care of AD patients currently.

55. What is memantine?

Memantine is a drug that works quite differently from the cholinesterase inhibitors. Memantine helps the action of **glutamate** that, like acetylcholine (discussed in Question 51), is a chemical compound secreted by nerve cells involved in learning and memory. Unlike cholinesterase inhibitors (discussed in Questions 52–55), memantine doesn't increase the amount of glutamate but causes it to work better. Patients both with mild to moderate AD and with advanced AD showed modest improvement after taking memantine. This is very important because cholinesterase inhibitors are not effective in the end stages of the disease. Patients in the advanced stage of AD have increasing problems with basic activities of daily living (e.g., difficulties in putting on clothing independently, difficulties with handling the mechanics of bathing and toilet use and, in some patients, difficulty in maintaining continence, discussed in Question 83). Performance of these tasks was modestly improved after taking memantine.

Glutamate

activating neurotransmitter abundant in the hippocampus and indispensable in the process of learning and making new memories.

Clinical studies did not demonstrate any greatly increased rate of side effects in AD patients in a group receiving memantine as compared to those in a group receiving placebo (a dummy substance without a drug). Also, memantine does not seem to interact very much with other drugs. This makes the use of memantine safe. The drug is produced by a German company, Merz Pharmaceutical, and has been available for several years in Europe. In the fall of 2003, the U.S. Food and Drug Administration approved memantine, and it's currently available for AD patients in the United States.

56. What are antioxidants?

Vitamin E and selegiline have antioxidant properties. As mentioned earlier, they can eliminate free radicals, which are poisonous by-products of certain reactions occurring naturally in your body. Free radicals are also greatly increased during inflammation. Increased production of free radicals has been thought to be associated with the development of AD. Selegiline (Eldepryl) is a drug initially developed to slow down the progression of Parkinson's disease, as increased production of free radicals has also been thought to be associated with this disease.

Studies have tested both vitamin E and selegiline in treating patients with AD. These studies have shown that neither vitamin E nor selegiline improve memory and cognitive test scores. What vitamin E or selegiline *can* do, though, is to increase survival in AD patients, lengthening the time before they require nursing home care and prolonging the time during which they're capable of performing activities of daily living (eating, grooming, or toileting). Vitamin E and selegiline seemed to be equally effective when used alone. Combining them didn't help any more than using either of them alone. On the basis of these studies, many doctors recommend the use of one antioxidant throughout the course of the disease. The dose of vitamin E used in these studies was 1,000 IU (international units) twice a day, and the dose of selegilin was 10 mg per day. Vitamin E is considered to be a "benign" medication, which means that most people can take it without side effects. Limitations exist for patients taking "blood-thinners," such as warfarin (Coumadin) and ticlopidine (Ticlid) because vitamin E has mild but established effects on bleeding. For such patients, starting and changing the dose of vitamin E needs to be conducted in connection with a physician prescribing therapy with blood-thinners.

Patients and caregivers also have to watch for bruises, and nasal and rectal bleeding. In turn, selegiline rarely can cause sleeplessness, psychosis, and agitation (discussed in Questions 73 and 75). Vitamin E is also less expensive than selegiline. In our practice, we tend to prefer vitamin E to selegiline.

57. Do cholesterol-lowering drugs slow the course of AD?

As mentioned, elevated cholesterol in midlife is a strong risk factor for developing AD after the age of 65 (discussed in Questions 10 and 20). Also, AD-transgenic animals develop more amyloid-β plaques when kept on a high cholesterol diet. If your total cholesterol or one of its subclasses is elevated above accepted limits, you should take drugs to lower its level. This will directly decrease your odds of heart attack, stroke, and related vascular dementia. If you have normal cholesterol, however, experts are unclear about whether you should take statins to lower cholesterol further, trying to stop the progression of AD, and to improve cognition. A clinical trial to investigate whether statins may slow the progression of AD is ongoing, and the results will be known within a year or two. Until the results of this trial are announced, no one can recommend taking statins for the treatment of AD.

58. Can hormone replacement therapy decrease AD symptoms?

Some uncertainty surrounds the impact of hormone replacement therapy on preventing AD (discussed in Question 49). Because evidence from animal experiments suggests that estrogen may improve memory, you may wonder whether regularly taking estrogen preparations may improve memory and cognition in the early stages of AD. Results from several studies testing the effect of estrogens on memory performance in early AD did not agree, but clearly they saw no large-scale improvement. Currently, the major drawback to estrogen therapy is that women who take estrogen are at a slightly higher risk for heart disease, blood clots, stroke, and breast cancer. Therefore, you should thoroughly discuss with your physician the pros and cons of taking this hormone. Hormone replacement therapy is not currently approved by the U.S. Food and Drug Administration for preventing or treating AD.

Some uncertainty surrounds the impact of hormone replacement therapy on preventing AD.

59. Can I take more than one drug for AD?

Yes, most of our AD patients are taking more than one drug for AD. The rule of thumb is to combine drugs with different routes of action but without adding to their side effects. Cholinesterase inhibitors (discussed in Questions 52–55) are currently the standard of care; therefore, most patients are taking either Aricept, Exelon, or Reminyl. We usually avoid combining two cholinesterase inhibitors because they would compete for the same target and at the same time multiply the chances of adverse effects.

A recent clinical trial demonstrated that patients taking both memantine and Aricept had better outcome than those in patients taking either memantine or Aricept alone. Because memantine and Aricept have clearly different routes of action, the cognitive benefits of these drugs can multiply without risk of increasing their side effects. Because memantine was recently approved by the U.S. Food and Drug Administration (FDA), more and more patients will be treated with memantine and cholinesterase inhibitors together.

In addition to taking one of the cholinesterase inhibitors, patients frequently take antioxidants (such as vitamin E). Although vitamins don't improve your memory or thinking process, they may slow down the progression of disease. Nothing prevents you from using selegiline as an antioxidant, but this drug is FDA-approved for treating Parkinson's disease only. Dietary supplements don't offer anything more than taking a cholinesterase inhibitor or vitamin E because most of these drugs work like a cholinesterase inhibitor (Huperzine A) or antioxidant (Ginkgo biloba or coenzyme Q10; all discussed in the following questions). Moreover, lack of quality control over available preparations questions their effectiveness and increases the chance of side effects.

ALTERNATIVE AND EXPERIMENTAL THERAPIES FOR AD

60. *What are alternative treatments for AD?*

Several herbal remedies and other dietary supplements have been promoted as effective treatments for AD and memory problems. If patients use an alternative medication, they have to realize several facts. First, claims about the safety and effectiveness of these products are based largely on testimonials, tradition, and a rather small body of scientific evidence. The U.S. Food and Drug Administration doesn't require rigorous scientific research for marketing dietary supplements as it does for prescription drugs. It has no authority over supplement production. It's a manufacturer's responsibility to develop and enforce its own guidelines for ensuring that its products are safe and contain the ingredients listed on the label and in the specified amounts. Also, bad reactions are not routinely monitored. Manufacturers are not required to report any problems that consumers experience after using their products. Second, dietary supplements can interact badly with prescribed drugs. Therefore, you shouldn't take any supplement without first consulting your physician. The following data cover a number of food supplements "recommended" for people with AD. Some of these supplements have been tested to lesser or greater extent in clinical trials.

Among all supplements related to AD, Ginkgo (an extract of the plant Ginkgo biloba*) is the best known.*

- *Ginkgo:* Among all supplements related to AD, Ginkgo (an extract of the plant *Ginkgo biloba*) is the best known. Ginkgo contains several compounds that may possibly have positive effects on cells within your brain and your body. Some think that Ginkgo extract may reduce the amount of free radicals and local inflation associated with the AD process in the brain. Some also think that Ginkgo can protect cell membranes and can regulate neurotransmitter function (discussed in Question 36). Ginkgo has been used for centuries in traditional Chinese medicine.

A small initial study in which participants were taking 120 mg a day of this extract demonstrated in some of them a modest improvement in cognition, activities of daily living (such as eating and dressing), and social behavior. The researchers found no measurable difference in overall cognitive impairment and memory test scores. Recently, The National Center for Complementary and Alternative Medicine of the U.S. National Institutes of Health launched a large, multicenter study to determine whether Ginkgo may help to prevent or at least delay the onset of AD or vascular dementia. Enrollment in this trial closed in 2002, and the trial will run for 5 years, so results will not be available until sometime after 2007. This multicenter trial involves 3,000 participants. Also, researchers are trying to uncover the exact methods by which Ginkgo works in the body. These studies are necessary to understand fully the potential therapeutic value of this supplement in treating AD.

Ginkgo has a few side effects that are somewhat similar to those of vitamin E. Ginkgo is known to reduce your blood's ability to clot; therefore, it's not recommended for use by people taking blood thinners (e.g., Coumadin or aspirin). Chances of internal bleeding from taking Ginkgo are unlikely but distantly possible. They increase with a lack of quality

Treatment

control of Ginkgo preparations. Other adverse effects include digestive tract irritation, allergic skin reaction, and headache.

- *Huperzine A:* Huperzine A is derived from the Chinese club moss, *Huperzia serrata,* a traditional Chinese herbal remedy used for centuries for treating fever, inflammation, and dementia. Evidence from small studies shows that the effect of huperzine A may be similar to that of approved cholinesterase inhibitor drugs (discussed in Questions 52–55). Huperzine A also has negative effects like those of cholinesterase inhibitors, including nausea, vomiting, and diarrhea. In addition, it significantly lowers your heart rate. Because huperzine A is a dietary supplement, it's unregulated and manufactured with no uniform standards.

    If you use huperzine A, you should monitor your condition for dangerous lowering of your heart rate. Therefore, if you're already taking medications that slow your heart rate (e.g., **beta blockers**) you shouldn't be taking huperzine A. Also, you shouldn't combine huperzine A with other inhibitors of acetylcholinesterase (e.g., Cognex, Aricept, Exelon, or Reminyl. Such a combination is unlikely to increase cognitive benefits, because both drugs would compete for this same path of action; however, the combination may multiply your chances of dangerous side effects.

- *Acetylcholine precursors:* As has been mentioned, AD patients lack acetylcholine, a chemical substance necessary for the function of nerve cells in the memory system. Because improvement can be obtained from giving AD patients cholinesterase inhibitors to decrease breakdown of acetylcholine, some have wondered about the possibility of

Beta blockers

heart medications used to slow heart rate and lower blood pressure.

increasing acetylcholine production. Nerve cells make acetylcholine from its precursor, lecithin. Therefore, some have suggested that extra intake of lecithin may boost acetylcholine production, thus reducing some of the symptoms of dementia. However, studies have shown that lecithin alone has little benefit over placebo (sugar pills) in improving cognitive performance in AD patients. Lecithin has also been used in combination with Cognex (tacrine), but it offered little additional benefit separate from Cognex.

- *Phosphatidylserine:* Phosphatidylserine is a form of fat that is the primary part of cell membranes in nerve cells. In those with AD and similar disorders, nerve cells die for reasons that are not yet understood. The strategy behind the possible treatment with phosphatidylserine is to shore up cell membranes and possibly protect those cells from dying. Early clinical trials with phosphatidylserine showed some promising result, although they recruited small numbers of participants. They were conducted using phosphatidylserine obtained from the brain cells of cows. This line of clinical investigations came to an end in the 1990s because of rising concerns about "mad cow disease." Some animal studies since then have attempted to see whether phosphatidylserine from soy may be a useful treatment. A small clinical trial showed modest benefit of phosphatidylserine from soy in 18 tested AD patients. A large carefully controlled trial is needed to test whether supplementing your diet with phosphatidylserine could be a viable treatment.

- *Coenzyme Q10:* Coenzyme Q10 is an antioxidant that occurs naturally in your body and is needed for normal cell reactions to occur. Its use to treat AD follows the same line of thinking as that for other antioxidants. A synthetic version of coenzyme Q10, called "idebenone," was tested for AD but did not show favorable results. Little is known about what dosage of coenzyme Q10 is considered safe, and you could experience harmful effects if you took it for a long period.

- *Melatonin:* Melatonin is a hormone involved in maintaining your day-sleep cycle. Its preparations are readily available as a remedy for sleeplessness. In addition, melatonin has antioxidant properties, like vitamin E, and in the test tube it shows some activity against the growth of amyloid-β deposits. Melatonin's effectiveness in preventing and treating AD has not been studied yet.

61. What is the vaccine for AD?

A real breakthrough in the development of potential therapies for AD was the invention of a vaccine that was shown to work successfully in transgenic mouse models of AD. Transgenic mice are genetically altered animals that can produce human amyloid-β (discussed in Questions 5, 12, 14, and 30). In other words, these are mice with an inserted human gene. Excess of amyloid-β in these transgenic mice leads to amyloid-β deposits in their brains similar to the condition found in early stages of AD in humans. In experiments performed in 1999, these mice received injections of an experimental vaccine that stimulated their immune system to produce antibodies against circulating amyloid-β in their blood. These antibodies were able to bind and clear circulating amyloid-β from their bloodstream so it couldn't go to their brain. Instead of going from blood into their brain, amyloid-β was going from their brain into their bloodstream. This resulted in clearing amyloid-β deposits in their brain and reversing the memory loss observed in these mice.

The vaccine was the first promising approach for treating AD by targeting the way in which the disease develops, not only offering mild temporary improvement. It offered a chance to halt the development of the disease. Promptly, researchers started clinical trials on humans. The first short trial on a few volunteers did not show that the use of vaccine in humans carried a potential for any dangerous negative effects. Immediately, researchers started a large clinical trial involving several hundred AD patients from many countries. Patients received their first dose of vaccine followed by booster doses about 3 months apart. Perhaps 1 year after the trial started, 18 patients displayed symptoms of brain inflammation, and one died after that. The trial was stopped for safety reasons. The researchers found evidence of disappearing amyloid-β plaques in the brain of the single person who died. Like transgenic mice, most vaccinated people generated antibodies against amyloid-β and showed a significant improvement in memory and cognition. This means that, although the vaccine may be associated with negative side effects in some, it can successfully target the ways in which AD works. Intensive research is under way to understand why in some people the vaccine caused brain inflammation and how this can be prevented in the future.

62. Will a better AD vaccine be available soon?

Liz's comment:

My husband is in the moderate stage of AD. He is seventy-six years old and he is in perfect physical shape. I realize that there is some risk related to the vaccine, but I would like to take it. Is there a possibility my husband can be vaccinated?

This is a question we encounter very frequently in clinical practice. Some people are willing to take the significant risk of brain inflammation, looking for hope in the cure of AD. The answer to this question, unfortunately, is no. Giving patients treatments that could harm them is illegal if such treatments haven't been approved by the U.S. Food and Drug Administration. The clinical trial of the vaccine for AD, although it was a failure, has proved that successful treatment for AD can be developed and that removal of amyloid-β from the bloodstream can reverse the routes by which amyloid-β piles up in the brain and can start clearance of AD plaques. New generations of vaccines are under development, in our own laboratory and those of a few others. Second-generation vaccine should meet two criteria: (1) to stimulate the immune system to produce antibodies against amyloid-b to help to clear it from the bloodstream and (2) to stimulate the immune system to limit its reaction to producing antibodies, not attacking the brain of treated individuals. Before the second-generation vaccine will be offered to humans, we have to perform extensive clinical trials on animals, including primates.

Researchers are also trying to develop alternative methods for removing excess amyloid-β from the bloodstream. Unlike the vaccine, by which your body would clear the excess of amyloid-β on its own, these approaches would require taking drugs on a constant basis. One of these approaches under development will be based on injections of antibodies that would target amyloid-β. Because antibodies have a limited life span, physicians would have to repeat your injections frequently. However, antibody injections are linked with fewer chances of encephalitis than is the use of the active vaccine. Other approaches are based on development of chemical compounds that would bind to amyloid-β and act as scavengers. Ideally, these compounds would be absorbed by the stomach, so they could be delivered in the form of pills and leave your body, with bound amyloid-β, through your kidneys with the urine or through the liver with bile.

At the moment, we provide Liz and people like her an explanation similar to that just described. We also offer her an option of putting her husband's name on the list so they may be called if and when the vaccine is available for clinical trial.

63. What is the shunt method of AD treatment?

The shunt is a device implanted by a brain surgeon, with one end located inside the skull and the other end in the heart or abdomen. The shunt is designed to remove an excess of cerebrospinal fluid (the fluid that cushions the brain; discussed in Question 31). A one-direction valve ensures that the fluid can be removed only from the brain, so backflow is not possible. This type of device is used to treat normal-pressure hydrocephalus (see Question 32).

Recently, researchers at Stanford University reported that experimental shunts had slowed AD progression in a small group of patients. This pilot study compared 12 patients, who had mild to moderate AD and had shunts implanted, with 11 AD patients, who received traditional care. After a year of monitoring and evaluation, the patients who had had the surgery remained stable while those who hadn't (called "control" patients) appeared to decline. Scientists don't understood the reasons why a shunt would stop AD progression, although those who performed the study couldn't see any adverse effect associated with the shunts. One has to remember that shunt implantation is a fairly major surgical procedure that's not free from severe risks. Ongoing research is trying to demonstrate shunt benefits and safety in a larger number of patients. Additional information on this study can be found at the following Web site: *www.eunoe-inc.com*.

PART FOUR

Caring for a Person with AD

How do patients tell other family members about a diagnosis of AD?

Why do people with AD become agitated?

What legal and financial issues I should be aware of?

More...

64. How does one tell other family members about a diagnosis of AD?

When they learn that they have diagnosed AD, many people hesitate to share this news with others. Some patients are afraid that disclosing their diagnosis may cause others to feel uncomfortable around them. However, it's important for them to talk to the people in their life about AD and about the changes they'll all experience together. AD is a long journey, not only for AD patients but for their significant others. Talking about the diagnosis is important for helping people to understand AD and to learn about how they can adjust to being a continuing part of others' lives.

You must understand that AD is not a normal part of aging but a brain disease that results in impaired (damaged) memory, thinking, and behavior and that these symptoms will progress over time. Patients must let family and friends be honest with how they feel about the diagnosis but should make it clear to them that although the disease will change all their lives, they want to continue enjoying the company of family and friends. AD patients will find that eventually it'll change many things in their relationships with family members and friends. Planning for these changes and talking about them honestly will help everyone.

You must understand that AD is not a normal part of aging.

PROGRESSION OF THE DISEASE

65. How do I adjust to changes in life in early AD?

AD will bring significant changes in day-to-day experiences. Things once done easily will become increasingly difficult. Here we have some suggestions to help you or your affected family member to cope with changes in daily life and how to be prepared for changes that will occur in the future. Because the most severe disability in the early stages of the disease concerns memory, we advise AD patients to support their memory with different types of reminders to limit confusion.

We frequently tell our patients to keep a book containing important information: phone numbers, people's names, appointments, and thoughts or ideas you want to hold on to. Most important phone numbers should be left in large print next to the phone. One of the family members or caregivers should prepare for the patient a schedule with things to do every day, such as meal times, regular exercise, a medication schedule, and bedtime. They should check the appropriate box once they've finished a given activity in the schedule. Patients must label their medications clearly and make sure that the old and outdated are discarded. The best option is to obtain a pill organizer. The easiest one is a pill box for all 7 days of the week, with three separate sections for each day: for morning, afternoon, and evening. Someone should supervise filling the pill box once a week; then it would be much easier to open one section at a given time of the day and take all necessary pills. Patients can also mark the days on a calendar to keep track of time and can label cupboards and drawers with words or pictures that describe their contents. They should keep closets and drawers neat and tidy, and avoid storing unnecessary items. Doing so will help them to find something when it's needed.

We frequently tell our patients to keep a book containing important information: phone numbers, people's names, appointments, thoughts or ideas you want to hold on to.

On the inside of the door, post reminders to turn off appliances and lock doors. Patients should always carry personal information, address, and contact phones to relatives when they're going out. When they go shopping, they shouldn't carry excess cash or more than one credit card. They should find somebody to supervise their finances, oversee bank statements, and balance their checkbook. They also may need somebody to do their major shopping and household chores. They can do difficult tasks during the times of the day when they normally feel best, should give themselves time to accomplish a task, and shouldn't force themselves or let others rush them.

Patients may also find communicating with others more difficult, both in understanding what people are saying and in finding the right words to express their thoughts. First make sure that their hearing is good. Many older adults may need a hearing device, which greatly improves communication. Ask the doctor about evaluating hearing problems. The test to evaluate hearing completely is called an **audiogram**. If patients have problems in communicating with someone, they should find a quiet place without distracting noise and take their time. They shouldn't be ashamed to ask someone to repeat a statement, speak slowly, or write down words if they don't understand.

Audiogram
a test to evaluate hearing.

Living alone may be very difficult for AD patients; however, many manage to do so in the early stage of the disease. They'll need some help from others. Also important is for their family to understand that they need extra help and that they have to mobilize some human resources. Their family has to appoint a trusted member to take charge of their financial resources (e.g., supervising bank accounts, paying utilities, and balancing the check book). This may require giving a trusted individual the legal authority (discussed in Question 91) to handle money matters. Checks, such as retirement pension or Social Security benefits, should be deposited directly in a patient's account. A patient may arrange for someone to help with house-keeping, meals, transportation, and other daily chores.

You can obtain information about assistance available in your community from your local chapter of the Alzheimer's Association or from your physician. A good recommended idea is always to have patients leave a set of house keys with a trusted neighbor. And the most important thing is to maintain as much social contact as possible. Therefore, have family and friends contact patients as often as possible, preferably at least once a day.

66. How does an AD patient cope with and adjust to family life after diagnosis?

The news of a diagnosis of AD is difficult to swallow. It's important, however, to understand that life isn't over. Living with AD means dealing with some life changes sooner than anticipated. The response of each person to a diagnosis of AD can be very different. People may exhibit a very broad range of emotions. Some people strongly deny the possibility of having dementia (discussed in Questions 27–29), and even many family members may deny the fact that their loved one is developing AD. The authors have encountered a number of cases in which family members (even some physicians) denied for a number of years that a relative had AD.

Many people experience anxiety and fear for the future. As the disease progresses, they may feel loneliness and frustration as they have difficulties in communicating and believe that no one seems to understand what they're going through. Inability to continue their professional career in many produces a feeling of loss and of personal worth. In many patients, these feelings trigger increased anxiety, problems with sleep (discussed in Question 71), and depression (discussed in Questions 37 and 40). Therefore, an awareness of depression and its treatment in early AD is extremely important. In addition to drug treatment of dementia, some measures may help them to take care of their emotional needs. First of all, they can't withhold their feelings; they should share them with friends and family. They can join a support group that they can locate through their local Alzheimer's Association chapter: *www.alz.org/ findchapter.asp*. Many may obtain comfort through contact with their clergy member. Some share feelings and experiences on-line at *http://www.alz.org/ ResourceCenter/Connections/ overview. htm*.

Remember, even if they're burdened with AD, patients can still continue a meaningful and productive life by taking care of their physical and emotional health, by engaging in activities they enjoy, and by spending time with their family and friends. They have to focus and get their family and friends involved to ensure the quality of their life for years to come. They shouldn't give up their hobbies but should try to stay active, exercise every day, and continue enjoying a social life on as many occasions as possible. Their endurance will be decreased, so they have to remember to rest when they're tired; they'll probably have to do this more often. They have to continue eating healthy food, with less fat and with more vitamins and fiber, and to reduce their alcohol intake. They must always take their medications and not skip regular visits to their doctor.

In adjusting to family life, remember that AD is a progressive process affecting not only AD patients but their families as well. As their ability to perform certain duties and activities declines, their spouse or other family members may have to take over these duties. What was once their responsibility in managing their household now becomes the responsibility of other family members. Because most people with AD continue to live at home even as the disease progresses, not only their household activities but their immediate care become the spouse's responsibility. The spouse may feel a sense of loss because of the changes the disease brings to their relationship. As the disease progresses, immediate caregivers often have feelings of tiredness and being worn out. Therefore, we highly recommend that they work with their spouse from the very beginning of the disease.

AD patients should not try to avoid household duties even if performing them comes with increasing difficulty. They should take their time and do them slowly, but not shift all the responsibility to their spouse. They shouldn't contribute to the feeling that now everything is on their spouse's head. Similarly, they should continue to participate in as many activities as they can, especially those they've always enjoyed. They must not avoid going out to the movies, theater, or restaurant. Remember that although the disease affects them, social stress related to the disease affects their spouse as well. They should try to give their spouse some feeling

Caring for a Person with AD

of normality. The need to try to continue to have a sexual life; if problems occur, they can seek professional counseling to discuss remedies. They must remember that their spouse is anxiously looking to the future regarding the progress of their disease. They can help to prepare for the future by working together on developing a long-term care plan. They should try to gather information together about caregiver services and their costs, such as housekeeping and respite care. They should encourage their spouse to attend a support group for caregivers and foster the feeling that they're concerned also about their spouse's health, including seeing a primary-care physician regularly.

The diagnosis of AD should not force patients to withdraw from contacts with other family members, who should also understand the meaning of changes brought by AD. They shouldn't avoid family meetings but try to maintain participation in family activities. Family members who are children and teenagers may find understanding AD-related changes particularly difficult. They may experience a wide range of emotions when they see that a grandparent is different. Some can be angry if they must take on more responsibilities. Some may feel embarrassed in front of their peers about their grandparent's behavior. AD patients shouldn't avoid children, nor should children avoid them. Younger children may need reassurance that the disease is not contagious and that although a loved one is sick, they can't "catch" AD. With older children and teenagers, patients and other adult family members need to remain straightforward about their memory and personality changes. It's natural for AD patients to forget grandchildren's names or say things that may embarrass them. They need to be assured that this isn't their fault or the AD patient's intention but that it is an effect of the disease. With their caregivers, AD patients can keep up with important events in the lives of their grandchildren and other younger relatives, such as birthdays, graduations, dating, or weddings.

67. What decision should AD patients make about their jobs?

Many professionally active people are given the diagnosis of mild cognitive deficit (memory defect only) or early AD. Such a diagnosis will require a certain adjustment in their professional life and prompt the need to plan for early retirement. Trying to conceal the diagnosis doesn't pay off: It is best to get the employer involved.

Those receiving a diagnosis of early-stage AD should discuss options with and try to get help from their employer. First they should talk about the diagnosis. Sometimes, providing educational materials or bringing someone with them to help explain their situation is helpful. They should continue to work as long as they, their employer, and their physician feel they're able. The other option is switching to a position that accommodates their limited abilities. They should try to remember that in the early stage of AD, learning new things may not be possible but that they can still use skills that they've learned before. Their routine and social skills remain unaffected. They may also think about reducing work hours.

When working, they should support their memory with all kinds of reminders and memos and a calendar. These changes may let them keep employment for a few years. They must realize, however, that sooner or later they'll have to retire. Therefore, they should try to research early retirement options. Once retired, they need to focus on finding activities to take the place of their job. They can consider volunteer work or a new hobby and stay as intellectually active as possible.

68. Can people drive a car if they develop AD?

The details of driving a car on busy roads demand quick reactions, alert senses, and making swift decisions. This becomes difficult for people with AD. A diagnosis of AD doesn't mean that you have to give up driving the moment the diagnosis is made. AD is a very prolonged process, and many people do quite well in the early stages of the disease. For many, restricting driving privileges means a loss of independence and mobility, often forcing people with the disease to rely on friends, family, and community services for transportation. Therefore, we recommend letting people with AD maintain their driving privileges as long as they are able to drive safely.

A diagnosis of AD doesn't mean that you have to give up driving the moment the diagnosis is made.

This in part depends on the conditions in which they do most of their driving. Driving on busy city streets with fast and aggressive traffic is quite different from slow, low-intensity suburban conditions. We recommend that caregivers regularly and closely monitor the safety of AD patients' driving. Several signs of unsafe driving should raise the red flag: failure to obey traffic signals, making slow or poor decisions, and driving at an improper speed. Caregivers should keep in mind that AD patients have impaired topographical memory (limited ability to recognize features that mark streets or exits), can't remember new routes, and may become lost easily in unknown surroundings. Therefore, they should be permitted to drive in a neighborhood they knew well before the onset of the disease. They shouldn't be allowed to drive in unknown surroundings or be expected to find a place according to verbal directions or a map. In such situations, they have to rely on others. Other warning signs of dangerous driving problems are episodes of uncontrolled rage, anger, or confusion while driving.

Persons with AD have to understand that at some future point they no longer can safely drive and that they'll have to surrender their driver's license and car keys. If you're a caregiver for such a patient and feel uncertain about the safety of continued driving, you may have the patient tested by the Department of Motor Vehicles. You may also ask a doctor for such an evaluation. Frequently, caregivers may encounter problems with an AD patient's unwillingness to give up car keys. You may ask a doctor to write a "Do not drive" prescription and substitute for the driver's license a nondriver photo identification card. If the AD patient continues attempts to drive or wanders off while driving, caregivers have to set strict limits on access to the car either by disabling it (removing the battery, for example) or by controlling access to the car keys. The nondriving transition may result in some anger and depression, which require understanding and sensitivity from caregivers and family. Caregivers should arrange for alternative transportation by involving other family members, friends, or community services.

The local chapter of the Alzheimer's Association may also provide transportation services to AD patients.

BEHAVIORAL SYMPTOMS AND ACUTE CHANGES IN MENTAL STATUS

69. Why do people with AD become agitated?

A number of behavior problems may be linked to AD. The word *agitation* is often used as an umbrella term to describe these behaviors. In the early stages of the disease, people with AD frequently experience personality changes, such as irritability, anxiety, or depression. These symptoms may be part of the way in which patients respond to their diagnosis and changes in life related to the early course of AD. Later during the disease, when cognitive deficits progress, patients may no longer be able to channel their energies into useful activities. As the result, AD patients may frequently begin pacing, constantly moving or being very restless. They may start purposeless activities: checking and rechecking door locks and appliances, tearing tissues, or playing with bed linen. Many patients experience emotional distress resulting from fear, frustration, and shame about their situation. They frequently utter verbal outbursts, using uncharacteristic cursing or threatening language, or they may even display violent behavior (discussed in Question 76). This kind of behavior produces emotional damage to caregivers. Caregivers may be frightened, upset, or simply exhausted by the demands and abuse of caring for a person who's agitated.

Because of their affected judgment and reasoning, AD patients often experience delusions (discussed in

Questions 72 and 73). Delusions are firmly held beliefs in things that aren't real. They may arise from fairly normal daily situations that healthy people usually disregard. Owing to their distorted view of a situation, AD patients may develop skewed meanings and believe things that aren't true. Among the most frequent delusions are beliefs that somebody is stealing from them. This often may arise from poor memory and confusion as to where objects were placed and how many were in their possession.

Advanced AD patients often have hallucinations (discussed in Question 72). The term *hallucination* is used to describe seeing, hearing, or feeling things that aren't present. People may often have hallucinations that result from mistaken views of things they notice around them and from affected judgment. Impaired hearing and vision, often linked to aging, contributes significantly to the frequency of hallucinations. Hallucinations often trigger and increase delusions in AD patients

Sleep disturbances (discussed in Question 71) are very frequent among AD and dementia patients. They especially struggle with problems in falling asleep. In the evening, they become more restless and agitated in what is called the "sun-downing" effect.

In most cases, episodes of agitation are a result of progressing disease. They may be triggered by many events in any situation, and caregivers have to be aware of these triggers. The pattern of behavioral changes in a given patient is usually similar, and caregivers are able to learn how to comfort and calm such patients. The treatment of agitation depends on a careful diagnosis and on identifying the triggers and types of agitated behavior taking place. Proper prevention, treatment, and intervention can often significantly lessen or stabilize the symptoms.

Caregivers have to be aware also that agitation and behavior changes may be signs of medical illness or drug interactions. In such cases, episodes of agitation are usually more violent and prolonged; caregivers aren't able to manage such patients as they usually do. In other words, the patient's behavior is strikingly different from that usually seen. This change in mental status is termed "acute" and requires prompt medical attention to find and remove its cause. The cause of such an acute change in mental status may be an infection (e.g., pneumonia or a urinary tract infection) or uncomforted pain. In some cases, prescription medication can cause agitation. This is most likely to occur when combined medications interact. Treating the underlying medical condition usually leads to a return to the baseline level of function.

70. How do I prevent and respond to agitation?

As a caregiver, you must understand what may cause bouts of agitation in AD patients so that you can actively prevent such episodes. You have to keep in mind that such patients adjust to and tolerate any changes in their surroundings poorly. Therefore, any significant change, such as remodeling a patient's room or switching rooms, travel to distant places, or change of a caregiver or home health aid may trigger an outburst. Occasionally, the presence of houseguests may be a trigger. Some patients may also respond with agitation when their caregiver tries to force them to take a bath or change clothing. Overstimulation by loud noises, an overactive environment, or physical clutter also often causes agitated behavior. One of the most common scenarios of when AD patients' behavior shows agitation and confusion is hospitalization. In this situation, in addition to being ill, the patient is placed all of a sudden in a very unfamiliar and uncomfortable place. This change often results in uncontrolled behavior. Unfortunately, this is a very common outcome seen in many hospitalized AD patients.

Several strategies can prevent or reduce agitated behavior in AD patients. They require a calm setting without stress, noise, glare, insecure space, and too much background distraction, including television. Caffeine use should be limited. All procedures should be simplified, and patients' routine and order should be maintained. AD patients cannot be challenged with difficult tasks; on the contrary, they should be offered a sense of security in what they are doing, stimulated only with gentle reminders and given frequent opportunities to rest.

You can try to identify signs of frustration, especially during such activities as bathing, dressing, or eating. Because advanced AD patients frequently have problems in making their needs known, you should check their personal comfort frequently for pain, hunger, thirst, constipation, a full bladder, fatigue, infections, and skin irritation. You have to make sure that they're in a comfortable temperature and are dressed adequately. During all these activities, you should respect their privacy. Dim lighting in a room greatly reduces the incidence of confusion and restlessness at night. A mandatory safety precaution is to remove firearms from a household where AD patients live (discussed in

Question 80). Also highly recommended is changing locks to a type that you can open from outside so patients can't lock themselves in.

As a caregiver, you need to know how to behave during an episode of agitation.

As a caregiver, you need to know how to behave during an episode of agitation. The right attitude is the best solution to an existing problem. Remember that judgment and reasoning of AD patients are limited. They may behave like children, with the difference that they don't have as much respect for your authority as children do. First, remain calm; don't raise your voice; don't criticize, ignore, confront, argue, demand, condescend, or force. Unfortunately, you have to endure the offense, but don't take their behavior personally. They aren't necessarily angry with you. They may have misunderstood the situation or be frustrated because of lost abilities caused by the disease.

Don't make sudden movements in AD patients' presence. Use calm positive statements that reassure them. Tell them they're safe and that everything is under control. Try to apologize even if the situation isn't your fault. Promise that you will stay until they feel better. You may use touch to reassure and comfort them. For example, put your arm around such a patient or give him or her a kiss. If necessary, calmly redirect their attention. If a patient is frustrated by, for example, failing to unbutton a shirt, use another activity as a distraction. After some time has passed, you can return to helping with unbuttoning the shirt. If despite what you're doing the situation gets out of hand, avoid using restraint or force. Unless the situation is extremely serious, don't try physical holding or restraint. That may cause more frustration and even cause personal harm. In such serious situations, you have to judge the level of danger—for both of you. You can often avoid harm by simply stepping back and standing away from a patient. If an AD patient is headed out of the house and onto the street, be more assertive. Luckily, this happens rarely. If an agitated patient becomes violent, simply step back and remain calm. In most situations, it doesn't take much time for such a patient to calm down.

71. How can I help with sleep problems?

Sleeping problems are present in roughly every fifth patient with AD. In the majority of cases, the symptoms clearly signal a syndrome called "late-day confusion" or "sundowning." AD patients experience periods of increased confusion, anxiety, agitation, and disorientation beginning at dusk and continuing throughout the night. These nighttime episodes of confusion and agitation require you to remain constantly alert and can interfere with your night's rest. Sundowning is one of the most common reasons for eventually placing AD patients in nursing homes. The reasons for sundowning are not clearly understood, but experts believe that it's related to a decreased need for sleep that's seen with aging and to disturbances of the day-night cycle caused by AD. Additional factors coming into play are affected judgment and difficulty in separating reality from the unreal. Therefore, AD patients function poorly in a room with reduced lighting and increased shadows. They may also have problems in separating dreams from reality when sleeping and waking. Sundowning problems are most common in the middle stage of AD and tend to disappear as the disease progresses.

As a caregiver you should be aware of a few things that can reduce the frequency of sundowning episodes. Try to plan active day schedules. Certainly try to avoid afternoon napping. Plan some activities, such as taking a walk, to make an AD patient more tired by the end of the day. Obviously, somebody who rests most of the day is likely to be awake at night. Restrict the eating of sweets and caffeine to the morning hours. If possible, completely avoid caffeine in the AD patient's diet. For those with a habit of drinking coffee, offer instant decaffeinated instead. Try to serve dinner early, and offer only a light meal before bedtime. Sometimes you can allow patients to sleep in a favorite chair or wherever they feel most comfortable. Remember also to keep the room partially lit; that's the best way to reduce agitation that's more likely to occur in dark or unfamiliar surroundings.

You should also mention sundowning episodes to the physician. Sometimes physical ailments, such as back pain when lying down or bladder or incontinence problems (discussed in Question 83), are contributing to sundowning. These problems can be treated and, in this way, the frequency of sundowning can be decreased. A doctor may also be able to prescribe medications to help an AD patient to relax at night. Many medications that AD patients take tend to have sedative properties.

One very simple solution that we prefer is to prescribe medications that have a sedative effect and are taken at night. For example, one of our AD patients also suffers from seizures. The dose of medication he took for seizures was divided, as in many other patients, into morning and afternoon doses to avoid sleeping during the day. When his daughter complained about sundowning, we changed the schedule, prescribing the entire dose in the evening. In this way, our patient did not have problems with sleep or with seizure control.

Even despite your biggest efforts, a patient may from time to time experience sundowning. If you suspect such a possibility, you should make sure that your home is safe and secure, especially if the patient wanders (discussed in Questions 84 and 85). Recommendations include limiting access to certain rooms or levels by closing and locking doors and installing tall safety gates between rooms. Door sensors and motion detectors can be used to alert family members when a patient is wandering. If you're awakened by a wandering, sundowning individual, avoid arguing or asking for explanations. Instead, remain calm and offer the reassurance that everything is all right and everyone is safe. Try to find out whether there's something bothering him or her or is needed. Offer a hug and gently point the way to bed.

72. Why do AD patients experience hallucinations?

Hallucinations are false notions of nonexisting objects or happenings. Hallucinations may affect all our senses. Visual hallucinations are commonly experienced by AD patients. They may report seeing the face of a former friend or people whom they used to fear. The latter is very common among AD patients who experienced the horrors of war. Hearing hallucinations involve hearing people's conversations or a single person's voice. Usually, the patients "hear" the voices of people they know saying innocuous phrases—never commands to take specific actions. This distinguishes

AD from other mental disorders, such as schizophrenia, with mainly hearing hallucinations that may govern patients' abnormal behavior. Less frequently, AD patients experience hallucinations from senses of touch (a feeling of being touched), smell (smelling odors not sensible to others), and taste (having a feeling of strange taste). The reason for AD patients' hallucinations is complex, but three major categories of problems can be distinguished. First, in the AD brain, the processing of various environmental stimuli delivered by different senses is affected; that's related to damage of nerve cells and loss of connections between them. Simply, AD patients may mistake a shadow for the face of somebody they knew in the past. Also, they have problems in separating what is taking place now from what occurred in the past. In normal persons, more recent events replace former experiences; AD patients who can't record new events may hang on to old memories more easily.

The second category of problems contributing to hallucinations are impairments of vision and hearing, which occur to a lesser or greater extent in the overwhelming majority of older people, not only in AD patients. Common visual problems (e.g., cataracts, glaucoma, macular degeneration, damage to the retina caused by diabetes) contribute to distortion of visual images which may then be misinterpreted by the ailing brain. **Presbyacousis**, an age-related hearing loss of higher tones, is also extremely common among older adults. Difficulties with hearing and with understanding somebody's voice in a noisy background are a part of this syndrome. In a noisy environment, AD patients may hear voices belonging to persons not present.

Presbyacousis

age-related hearing loss, especially to higher-frequency sounds (e.g., a kettle whistle), which is extremely common in the elderly and helped by use of a hearing aid.

The third reason for hallucinations is medications. Older adults may have multiple health problems and may take a number of medications for heart, diabetes, cancer, and other conditions. Some of these medications, especially those with a tendency to build up in the system, may cause various forms of hallucinations as a negative effect. This type of problem is more likely to occur in AD patients or in those with other types of dementia than in normal-thinking adults. If the hallucinations occur randomly, you may choose to ignore them; however, if they start to happen more frequently, you should discuss them with the patient's physician. The physician should try to determine their likely cause by examining the patient for problems with vision and hearing, by performing blood tests, and by reviewing the patient's medications list to see whether any are likely to cause hallucinations. The rate of visual and auditory hallucinations sometimes can be greatly decreased by simple measures (e.g., prescribing glasses or a hearing aid or withdrawing one offending drug). In other instances, ophthalmological (eye) surgery or treatment may help.

Although these measures may decrease the frequency of hallucinations, many people with AD may still experience them at times. The hallucinations may result in periods of fear, but they may also trigger episodes of agitation and delusions.

You as a caregiver can take a few simple measures in response to hallucinations and to prevent their occurrence. If patients report seeing or hearing something that's obviously a hallucination, respond in a calm, supportive manner and offer assurance. Try to distract them from paying attention to the hallucination by bringing attention to you. Either grab their hand or tap a shoulder. Try to avoid arguing about what is seen.

Caring for a Person with AD

Try to share their fear and ask about feelings behind the hallucinations, whether they're worried or frightened. Distract their attention from the content of the hallucinations by starting a conversation or bringing them to another room, preferably well lit and occupied with other people. Remember: Unclear background noises, darkness, and being alone fuel hallucinations in AD-affected patients. Try to pay attention to these factors and eliminate them as much as possible.

73. What are paranoia and delusions?

Delusions are false beliefs not shared by others. They tend to be maintained firmly, even when they don't agree with reality. Paranoia is a complex system of delusions that directs an AD patient to act. Common examples of delusions among AD patients are delusions of infidelity, **erotomania**, and feelings of being persecuted, being poisoned, or being robbed. These strange beliefs result from impaired judgment and abstract thinking, loss of control of social rules, and poor orientation and memory. Delusions and paranoia are frequently built on minor daily events that otherwise are considered meaningless. For example, AD patients who tend to misplace objects may start to believe that some objects, including valuables, are being stolen from them. A caregiver who confronts them finds these valuables located in an unusual place. If after such a discovery such patients refuse to acknowledge that no theft took place, the idea starts to become a delusion. This may grow to full paranoia when such patients lock themselves inside their house—afraid of thieves—and don't let anybody in.

Erotomanic delusions may start with believing that a teenager from a house across the street may be a secret

Paranoia is a complex system of delusions that directs an AD patient to act.

Erotomania
excessive interest and preoccupation with sexual matters that may be associated with AD or other forms of dementia as a result of destroying parts of the brain responsible for controlling and suppressing urges and impulses.

lover, so such patients start to write and send out love letters. The most common infidelity delusion (belief in an unfaithful spouse) among AD patients is that a spouse has a younger lover. During the development of this paranoia, such patients may want to arrange for a divorce or may request a lawyer to change their living will. Because the spouse is most frequently the closest caregiver and the one who is the most emotionally affected by the disease of their beloved, such infidelity delusions and paranoia may cause great emotional suffering.

Similarly, erotomanic delusions may result in social consequences, and the described delusions of stealing and locking oneself inside the house may lead to physically dangerous situations. Some people reading this book may consider the description of these different beliefs to be very far-fetched, but this type of behavior may turn life into a horror for many families whose members with AD suffer from these delusions and paranoia.

Delusions are most common in early and middle stages of AD. Sometimes they may show up in cognitively normal older adults who have not had such symptoms before. In many cases, so-called geriatric or late-life paranoia may be a symptom that announces the start of AD.

74. What is Capgrass syndrome?

Capgrass syndrome is seen in advanced dementia and is a form of delusion. An example is seen in AD patients who deeply believe that a family member (e.g., a son or a daughter or a spouse) is not their son or daughter or spouse but is a fraud. You can imagine how this situation must be difficult and frightening for loving caregivers.

Capgrass syndrome
belief by a person with advanced dementia that relatives are imposters.

The causes of Capgrass syndrome are not fully understood. One theory suggests damage to the amygdala, a part of the brain that's very close to the hippocampus and is involved in processing emotions and learning ties between facts, faces, pictures, and emotions. For example, thanks to the amygdala, children learn to connect a picture of a mother's face or silhouette with feelings of love and safety. Later on, each time these children encounter a mother's picture, they recall these good memories. Parents develop these same relationships among voices, faces, pictures, and warm emotions toward their children. In AD patients, the amygdala is damaged; therefore, seeing their relative's face may not produce the related normal feelings. Such patients' subconscious explanation may be that this is not their child or spouse, although they appear to be the same; therefore, it has to be an impostor. Because in persons with advanced AD the brain's capacity is limited, they may act weirdly on these false beliefs by being aggravated and agitated, requiring treatment with **antipsychotic medications**. In many cases, such patients improve under treatment, and their symptoms subside.

Antipsychotic medications

class of medication used to treat psychosis, delusions, and agitation in AD patients.

75. Can agitation and behavioral symptoms be treated medically?

The first-line treatment of agitation is a behavioral approach: recognizing and avoiding the factors triggering the agitation. You as caregiver also have to know how to respond in a case of agitation (discussed in Questions 69 and 70). In some instances, behavioral approaches don't work, and patients may require drug treatment. Many different things may cause agitation in AD patients; a physician prescribing medication has to examine and address such things. Physicians also have to judge whether symptoms of depression or delusions and paranoia (or both) cause agitation episodes.

What you as caregiver also have to remember is that drugs for agitation and behavioral symptoms have to be given on a regular basis, usually once a day. These drugs aren't going to work when they're administered for just a one-time event. Drug treatments usually reduce the frequency and severity of symptoms but rarely get rid of them completely. You still have to remember that medications are most effective when they're combined with changes in behavior or surroundings. What follows is a short review of drugs used to treat agitation and behavior symptoms, together with the most common side effects you should be aware of. In general, treatment of agitation and irregular behavior begins with a single drug at low doses

Antidepressants work especially well in treating symptoms of agitation connected with low mood, irritability, or depressed appetite. The antidepressants most often prescribed for AD patients belong to a group called **serotonin reuptake inhibitors** because they increase the amount of a brain chemical called **serotonin**. Examples of these drugs are Celexa (citalopram), Prozac (fluoxetine), Paxil (paroxetine), and Zoloft (sertraline). They are usually administered once a day and have few possible side effects (abdominal cramps, diarrhea, constipation, nausea, and rare vomiting). These symptoms usually aren't serious and don't last long. Serotonin reuptake inhibitors may increase bleeding time, so they should be avoided around the time of planned surgery.

Some patients respond well to **anxiolytics** (anxiety reducers), such as Ativan (lorazepam) or Serax

Serotonin reuptake inhibitors

class of medication used to treat depression by increasing levels of serotonin.

Serotonin

neurotransmitter that when lacking is associated with symptoms of depression (e.g., low mood, excessive feeling of guilt, slowness, changes in sleep and eating habits).

Anxiolytics

class of medication used to treat anxiety and agitation.

(oxazepam). They're usually administered in small doses and treat anxiety and agitation. These medications given in the evening have sedative properties and may help with sleep problems (discussed in Question 71).

Delusions and paranoia (discussed in Question 73) should be treated with antipsychotic drugs, such as Zyprexa (olanzapine), Seroquel (quetiapine), Clozaril (clozapine), or Risperdal (risperidone). They're used to treat many psychiatric diseases that cause delusions but, for older adults with AD, they're usually prescribed in much lower doses. In addition, these drugs can treat hallucinations (discussed in Question 72), aggression, and hostility and can help with uncooperativeness. Antipsychotic drugs can produce negative effects, so-called **extrapyramidal symptoms.** These include acute stiffening of muscles in the body, restlessness (a constant need to pace or to fuss with objects), and involuntary movements of facial muscles and the hands. Although any antipsychotic drug can trigger these side effects, in practice Zyprexa, Seroquel, and Clozaril are the safest. Seroquel and Clozaril are often used to treat side effects caused by other antipsychotic drugs. Also, Clozaril may cause damage to the bone marrow, so blood counts have to be checked on a monthly basis.

Extrapyramidal symptoms

a group of symptoms including stiffening of the body, involuntary movements, restlessness, and tremor.

76. What can I do if an AD patient develops severe mental status changes?

A severe change in mental status is a medical emergency and requires prompt medical handling in a hospital emergency room. The quality and circumstance of a mental status change greatly depends on the stage of the patient's AD. Patients may experience an episode of confusion (sometimes linked to agitation; discussed in Questions 69 and 70) and irrational behavior on a level not noticed before. Then again, they may not respond to the usual approaches used by caregivers or may become withdrawn and interact poorly. The first situation, called **delirium**, is more likely to occur in the early and middle stages of AD; the second is more common in advanced stages of the disease. What follows are examples of such behavior.

Delirium
acute change in mental status associated with irrational behavior and agitation.

Anna's comment:

My mother, who is 82 and has moderate AD, lives with us. She's still able to help me with household chores, but she's unable to perform more complex tasks, like planning a dinner for a number of people and doing the shopping. When I'm at work, she goes to a senior citizen center every day for dinner. She locks the apartment door after herself and goes to a place one block down the street. She usually returns two hours later. This time, when I came back from work, she wasn't at home. After an extensive search, I found her in a neighboring park. She was confused. She was able to recognize me but not our neighbor, and she was unable to answer questions about her home address. When she was brought to the emergency room, she became more agitated and combative. When examined by a doctor, she did not follow commands and was unable to answer a number of simple questions that she usually would answer.

Mary's comment:

My aunt is 79 and has end-stage AD; she lives with us but requires twelve hours a day home aid. She walks with a walker and follows most simple commands. Her verbal output is limited to simple sentences. She can ask for what she needs. She smiles. She's unable to dress herself or take care of her toilet needs.

Today, as I was leaving for work, she seemed to be less alert than usual, but I thought she was a little bit sleepy. When I came back in the evening, my aunt was lying in her bed with eyes open, but she did not respond to my questions. When I put my fingers on the palm of her hand, she grasped my hand spontaneously. The home health aid said that she refused to get up from the bed since morning,

What is the cause of an acute change of mental status in AD patients? Degenerative diseases (such as AD) leave the brain oversensitive to stress related to many processes, such as infection going on somewhere in the body, **electrolyte** imbalance, or toxic side effects of drugs. We all get infections from time to time, such as colds or flu, and take drugs without changing our mental status. However, the AD brain has diminished tolerance to such conditions. Medical evaluation in a hospital revealed that Anna's mother suffered from a urinary tract infection, whereas Mary's aunt had the beginning of pneumonia. Both patients were admitted to hospital and were treated with intravenous antibiotics. In addition, physicians gave Anna's mother mild antipsychotic drugs because at first her confusion and combativeness increased because of her unfamiliar hospital ward surroundings.

The list of possible causes of severe mental status changes in AD patients is long, starting with various kinds of infections (e.g., urinary tract infections, pneumonia, bronchitis, **otitis** [ear inflammation] from interactions of medications) or age-related damage to kidney or liver functioning. As you can see, these processes are primarily located outside the brain. Inflammation of the brain or **meninges** (membranes surrounding and cushioning the brain), brain tumor,

Electrolytes

general name for a number of ions (e.g., sodium, calcium, potassium, and others) that have to be maintained at an appropriate level in the serum. Changes in serum levels of certain metabolites may cause seizures or a change in mental status.

Otitis

ear inflammation.

Meninges

membranes surrounding and cushioning the brain.

seizures, or stroke may also cause changes in mental status, but these conditions are relatively rare. As has been said, severe mental status changes are clearly different from occasional agitation caused by, for example, bathing. Remember, severe changes are a medical emergency and require immediate medical attention. The extent of this testing (discussed in Questions 40–45) should include general physical and nervous system examinations, complete blood and urine tests, chest x-ray, brain computed tomography, and often a lumbar puncture. Because medications can cause mental status changes, we always strongly encourage caregivers to keep an updated list of all drugs being taken and their dosages together with the diagnoses and phone numbers of treating doctors. Providing such a list to emergency room staff will help greatly in coming to the correct diagnosis swiftly. Treatment is based on removal of the offending cause, as in treating an infection in the two described examples.

Remember, severe changes are a medical emergency and require immediate medical attention.

What has to be mentioned also is that AD patients may have lengthy mental status changes after any major surgery (e.g., heart surgery or hip replacement). Toxic and metabolic stress related to surgery causes such changes, and use of narcotic painkillers in addition can increase the effect. Even when no other complication occurs, it takes a little bit more time for AD patients to return to their previous condition after any procedure.

77. Do dementia patients often have seizures?

Unfortunately, yes. Seizures (fits or convulsions) are frequent among persons in the advanced stages of AD and also affect every fourth person who has had a stroke (discussed in Question 12); this includes patients with vascular dementia (discussed in Question 30). Several types of seizure may exist in patients with dementia. One is associated with generalized shaking: Such patients typically fall to the floor, and their entire body (including their head and extremities) shakes. Severe injuries (e.g., bone fractures) may result from such a fall. Generalized seizures last usually less than a minute. Passing urine is frequent, and passing feces can happen (discussed in Question 83). Patients who have had these generalized seizures remain in a state of deep sleep for a period of minutes to a few hours. Generalized seizures may also happen when AD patients are asleep. The noise of convulsions usually brings a caregiver's attention to such events.

Complex partial seizure

form of seizures associated with impaired consciousness.

Focal seizures

form of seizures associated with uncontrollable shaking of one limb or half of the body while a patient usually remain conscious.

Electroenceph-alogram

recording of electrical activity of the brain, used to detect and characterize seizures.

A less severe form of seizures is called **complex partial seizures**. These are periods of limited unresponsiveness during which patients may fall to the ground, but they may also remain in a sitting or (rarely) even in a standing position. During such a seizure, patients can't speak (but may make nonverbal noises) and don't respond to commands or to voices. These attacks last less than a minute, although rarely they may continue for as long as several hours. The least harmful and least frequent form of seizure is called **focal seizures**. They produce uncontrollable shaking of one limb or half the body, with the patient remaining normally responsive.

The first episode of seizure, regardless of its type, is a medical emergency and typically requires a patient's admission to hospital for evaluation. The medical checkup usually includes an **electroencephalogram** (recording electrical activity of the brain) and a magnetic resonance image (MRI). The latter is to exclude a tumor, bleeding, or infection that may cause seizures.

A patient who has a neurodegenerative disease and once had a seizure is likely to have more similar episodes and has to be given antiseizure drugs, called **anticonvulsants**. Numerous anticonvulsants are available to treat patients with dementia and seizures. The general rule is to prescribe anticonvulsants that don't have an impact on patients' mental status. Successful treatment with anticonvulsants should ensure that seizures don't happen again. Patients need, however, to take the medication regularly every day without exception. Most anticonvulsants also require checking their level in the blood. Some can be harmful to patients' bone marrow or liver, so suitable blood tests have to be scheduled every 3 to 6 months.

Anticonvulsant
medication given to stop or prevent seizures.

CARING FOR A PATIENT WITH ADVANCED AD

78. How do I live day by day with an AD patient?

AD is a progressing disease, increasingly limiting activities performed independently. Patients entering the later stages of the disease require more and more support to survive. A proper system of support is based on the availability of caregivers, who have to take over more and more tasks. Most often, AD patients' spouses become the primary caregiver, and the weight of household responsibilities falls on their shoulders. Unfortunately, caring for AD patients requires a lot of attention, effort, and time. At first, caregiving mainly concerns financial matters and paying bills, but later it includes cooking, cleaning, shopping, and (eventually) dressing and personal hygiene. For AD patients, you as a caregiver can make a big difference between their feeling needed and loved and feeling unnecessary and unloved.

Although you have a much greater burden of responsibility, you should try to incorporate AD patients into your daily activities as much as possible. You can start this process by answering several questions:

- What skills do such patients still have, and what activities can they still perform?
- Can they begin and perform these activities without direction and supervision?
- What activities can they enjoy doing?

Thinking about these questions, you may quickly realize that even people in the middle stage of AD may still perform and enjoy a lot of household activities (e.g., helping with cleaning, cooking, laundry, or gardening). Patients not only enjoy doing these tasks, they have the chance to interact with other human beings. When you involve patients in these activities, you have to focus on enjoyment and interaction, not on achievements. You may offer support, supervision, and simple instructions. AD patients perform activities best as a part of daily routine. The best option is for you to try to structure the day by combining activities related both to patient care and to maintaining the household.

You should start the day by supervising AD patients with daily hygiene and dressing. Try to involve them in preparing breakfast, eating the breakfast together, and cleaning up together after breakfast. During breakfast, you may discuss papers, books, news regarding family, and photos. Household duties usually require going out (e.g., to do shopping). You can do this together. You should show patients that you enjoy their company. Of course, you'll accompany them to the doctor but, in addition, they can accompany you as well when *you* go for your routine medical checkup. In the afternoon, you may prepare and eat dinner together, wash dishes, and go for a walk. In the evening, you can watch TV or listen to music together. At the end of the day, you may supervise the patient's bath and going to bed.

As you see, the need is for spending time together. You may be sure that AD patients will enjoy time spent and conversations with you. You probably realize that they have difficulties both with understanding others and with expressing themselves. They speak less often because they sometimes have difficulty in finding the right words, especially those that are difficult. Use familiar words repeatedly and rely on unspoken gestures. They may also have difficulties in organizing words logically, so frequently they lose their train of thought. Such limits require special habits to make mutual communication stress-free and enjoyable. Try to speak clearly and slowly, maintain eye contact, and use short, simple, familiar words. When you're supervising patients, try to give instructions in small, clear, simple steps. Don't ask more than one question at a time and allow enough time for a response. Spending time with AD patients and involving them in daily activities not only can make life for both of you more enjoyable but can greatly reduce their anxiety and episodes of agitation.

79. How do I get other family members involved in care?

Some caregivers try not to accept assistance from others and attempt to handle everything themselves. Unfortunately, this may cause them to become burned out, depressed, and resentful toward their AD-affected loved ones. Asking others for assistance is not a sign of weakness or failure, and patients can only benefit if the efforts of several caregivers are pulled together. Then again, family members withdraw from interacting socially with AD patients and their caregiver. That's because they don't understand the changes brought on by the disease and are afraid of patients' strange behavior. Family members may also deny what's happening or may disagree about financial and care decisions. Establishing durable power of attorney and a living trust (discussed in Questions 91 and 92) can clarify who is to make these decisions. Sometimes, calling a family meeting helps.

During the family meeting, you should be open regarding your feelings as a caregiver. Talking about caregiver roles and responsibilities, problems, and feelings can help to ease tensions. In many situations, providing education about the disease and its symptoms and the tasks of a caregiver have helped to break barriers. Also helpful is to invite a professional counselor or clergy member to participate in such a meeting.

Involve other family members in caregiving duties. You can share the caregiving responsibilities by making a list of tasks, including how much time, money, and effort may be involved to complete them. Tasks have to be divided according to family members' preferences and abilities. You should learn to acknowledge interpersonal differences. Some people may volunteer, responding immediately to issues and organizing resources; others may feel comfortable with being told to complete specific tasks. In many cases, AD affecting one family member results in a divided family. A family meeting designed to unite efforts in caring for that patient may be a first step to bring the family together.

In many cases, AD affecting one family member results in a divided family.

This communication has to be extended for regular family meetings or conferences to keep the family up to date on patient care issues and to decide whether to make any changes in responsibilities. You and other family members may also realize that you enjoy doing a number of activities together as a family while involving the patient. Examples of such activities are common walks, listening to music, watching a movie, looking at old photographs, making a family tree, or doing household chores.

80. What home changes will make it safer for a patient with advanced AD?

For various reasons already described, AD patients are prone to accidents, some of which may happen while inside the house. If you're caring for an individual with AD at home, you should change some things to make the environment safer. Because these patients are easily disoriented and confused—especially in dark rooms and corridors—their living area should be well lighted. Colored contrasting rugs placed in front of doors or steps may help patients to anticipate staircases and room entrances. Similar tricks can be used to point the way to the bathroom. To mark the entrance to the patient's room, a small picture or favorite photos can be hung on the door. To prevent patients from locking themselves inside a room, by choice or by accident, you should change the locks of inside doors to nonlocking knobs. This especially applies to such places as bath-rooms, bedrooms, and the basement. You have to put locks on doors to bar access to places where possibly dangerous things are kept (e.g., appliances, furnaces, chemicals, cleaning fluids, sharp tools, electrical tools, lawn mowers, or knives).

Caring for a Person with AD

AD patients' access to firearms is not acceptable. You have to lock both hand guns and hunting rifles in a safe box. To limit the possibility of wandering (discussed in Questions 84 and 85), you should install deadbolts on the entrance door and the door to a backyard. You can equip these doors additionally with a remote alarm that sounds in a distant house section when that door has been opened. You can also check wandering by using a motion detector with a remote alarm.

Because AD patients are given to falls that can often result in serious injuries (including fractures), you have to take certain measures to prevent them. This includes removing objects, such as floor lamps, magazine racks, furniture containing glass parts, and other obstacles; installing handrails; and making sure that floors are not slippery. Because many accidents happen in bathrooms, install walk-in showers, put a nonslippery mat on the floor, and install grab bars.

Other safety issues may require you to supervise an AD patient strictly in taking prescription and over-the-counter drugs; in smoking and alcohol consumption; and in regularly cleaning out the refrigerator and discarding inedible food. Preparing the house for the safe care of an AD patient should also include being prepared for various kinds of emergencies. Try to keep an updated list of emergency phone numbers and addresses for local police and fire departments, hospitals, and poison control help lines. Also, regularly check the fire extinguishers and smoke alarms. Making all these changes means a lot of work. Realistically, some of them are not applicable to every household.

You have to weigh their usefulness for ensuring safety against limiting a patient's independence.

81. How do I manage an AD patient's personal hygiene?

As AD progresses, patients tend to lose their ability to maintain personal hygiene, and they cease to care about obvious flaws in their appearance. At some point, they start to require daily help and supervision in the most basic and routine tasks. This kind of assistance is sometimes very problematic because it often requires you to invade their privacy, which may trigger episodes of agitation and outbursts of aggression (discussed in Questions 69, 70, and 76). Depending on their stage of disease, AD patients can have difficulties in dressing. First, they tend to wear the same clothing every day and don't pay attention to whether they're clean or dirty and torn. Then, they have problems in dressing in the correct order; eventually, they may not be able to put their clothes on and zip or button them.

Maintaining a satisfactory physical appearance contributes to our sense of self-esteem. When you help AD patients with dressing, you have to consider their likes and dislikes. Although you have to make some compromises so that the dressing process is simpler and less time-consuming, what's important whenever possible is to combine patients' past routine and style with the current one. You'll have to prepare a set of clothing for them every morning, but try to give them a sense of making their own decisions by offering two or three choices of shirts, pants, and sweaters. You'll also have to organize the process of dressing for them.

Put particular pieces of clothing in front of them (e.g., spread on a bed, in the order in which they need to be put on). You can hand patients one piece after another with short, simple instructions. Be calm, don't rush or reprimand them, because that may only result in agitation and anxiety. Because AD patients often want to wear the same outfit day after day, try to get several of the same or slightly different articles so that they can always wear a clean and neat set. The garments you choose should be comfortable and easy to put on and take off. Shirts that button in the front and cardigans are easier to handle than pullover tops. Patients would prefer Velcro to zippers, buttons, and snaps. Shoes have to be comfortable and easily pulled on and off, but they must not cause patients to fall, so avoid slip-on shoes or sandals.

Patients with advanced AD may find that maintaining proper dental hygiene is difficult. Not only may they cease to care about this need; they may have difficulties with brushing or flossing their teeth. Patients who are told "brush your teeth" may simply not do it because this task is beyond their abilities. You can achieve better results by simplifying tasks (e.g., handing them a toothbrush with toothpaste on it and guiding their hand to start the process). You have to oversee their oral care daily. Flossing may be too difficult for AD patients, so you have to do it. Also, you have to make sure that their dentures are removed in the evening and placed in a labeled container. You also have to check dentures for cracks and inspect their mouth for pressure sores. We recommend that AD patients see a dentist for a checkup every 4 to 6 months.

Bathing is a very private part of personal hygiene. It may also be the most challenging task you have to face. Patients with advanced AD may regard bathing as an extremely unpleasant experience often linked to feeling cold. They also do not appreciate the need for personal hygiene. Therefore, you may often encounter agitated and disruptive behavior (discussed in Questions 69 and 70), such as screaming or even hitting. Because arguing and use of force won't produce any results, you have to be patient and gentle. First, you can make sure that they're not feeling cold by raising the room temperature and carefully adjusting the water temperature. Don't rush them and don't make them feel overwhelmed with the situation. Be gentle, especially with their hair; avoid scrubbing, scratching, and pulling.

Many AD patients still remain self-conscious about nakedness. Let them hold a towel in front of their body and keep a robe nearby. At all times in the bathroom, don't forget the possibility of a fall. Place a non-slip mat on the floor and in the bathtub, and attach grab bars to the walls. Also, proper hygiene doesn't mean that patients have to take a bath every day.

82. How can I avoid embarrassing situations?

The judgment of AD patients is known to be distorted. This may produce a number of unpredictable situations that may put a spouse, other family members, and caregivers in an awkward position. Although some of these situations may be taken with humor, others are really embarrassing because the behavior involved doesn't match the patient's previous social status and position. To avoid such behavior, try to identify its cause so that in the future you can come up with possible solutions to prevent a repeat. Bold sexual behavior is an example of such a situation. AD patients may forget that they're married and may begin to flirt or make inappropriate advances toward members of the opposite sex. They may also disregard the fact that their target is married and may take such actions publicly. To interrupt this awkward situation, try to distract them with another activity. Unload the weight of the problem by apologizing to the person put in that awkward situation and explain the medical nature of the problem. Try to bring such patients into a private place and slowly—without emotion—explain that the action is incorrect. If such patients are married, explain that this behavior isn't going to make their spouse happy. Although AD patients may lack judgment and the ability to curb certain urges, they're still sensitive to criticism and may feel as ashamed as any normal person. Try to act gently, and avoid becoming angry or laughing at the person.

Other examples of socially unacceptable and embarrassing behavior may be public criticism of how other people dress or behave or of what they're saying. Sometimes we don't agree with other people's points of view, but social manners prevent us from direct public criticism. Because in AD patients these drives may not be properly channeled and curbed, they may criticize other people in a public situation, and it may even lead to aggressive exchanges. You may find avoiding this behavior more difficult than that of bold sexual advances. Interrupt such patients' behavior by distracting them. Don't contradict their opinions, admit their rights, but try to emphasize that publicly attacking other people is wrong.

Shoplifting is another common embarrassing situation committed by AD patients. They may not understand or remember that merchandise must be paid for, so they may casually walk out of a store without paying for something—unaware of any wrongdoing. When they're caught by shop staff, such patients usually feel very embarrassed. Providing patients with a wallet-size card explaining that they have AD may be helpful, but if this behavior continues, it means that they need constant supervision when shopping.

As described in Question 78, dressing problems are common in AD patients. They may tend to wear the same clothing over and over, may not care about the condition of that clothing, or may dress in the wrong order. AD patients also have difficulties with expressing their needs. If a piece of clothing isn't comfortable, they may instead simply take it off in public, unmindful of the results. A measure to prevent this type of behavior is to make sure that clothing they wear is comfortable.

AD patients also have difficulties with expressing their needs.

In Question 73, we discussed paranoia and delusions in AD patients. This type of behavior often leads to conflicts and embarrassing situations. Delusions of a spouse's infidelity and stealing by family or servants are typical and may result in false, psychologically damaging charges. Drug treatment of paranoid and delusional behavior (discussed in Questions 49–55) may decrease its frequency and likelihood but may not remove such a possibility completely. In cases of paranoia, don't openly argue with patients; rather, try to distract their attention. Reassure them that everything is all right, that everybody loves them, and that nothing wrong is going to happen.

83. How do I deal with incontinence in an AD patient?

People in advanced stages of AD experience loss of bladder control followed by loss of bowel control. This mainly comes from losing the so-called "toilet reflex," a trained behavior that we learn in childhood. It allows us to withhold the need to urinate or defecate until it can be performed in the right conditions. However, numerous treatable medical conditions also may contribute to incontinence. If they're handled correctly, eliminating them may decrease the chance for unwanted incidents. In the case of urinary incontinence, a new urinary tract infection has to be ruled out as being a cause. Some gender-specific conditions may often contribute to incontinence (e.g., prostate enlargement, in men and weak pelvic muscles in women). Strain, sneezing, laughing, or coughing may trigger incontinence. Some people take drugs, called **diuretics**, to increase their urine volume. These drugs are taken for many medical reasons, such as hypertension, but you may ask the patient's prescribing physician to replace the diuretics with another category of drug if urinary incontinence is a problem. Also, drinking excessive amounts of fluids, in particular those with caffeine (e.g., coffee, soda, and tea, all of which have diuretic properties), should be avoided. Try to decrease AD patients' intake of tea and coffee in general, and try to decrease the amount of fluids they drink in the latter part of the day. This may help with incontinence at night.

Diuretics

medications used to increase urine output and used to treat hypertension and heart and kidney failure.

For a certain number of patients, incontinence occurs on their way to the bathroom. Try to modify their environment to make sure that they have no trouble in finding the bathroom or getting to it in time. Sometimes, providing visual clues, such as a bright rug on a corridor leading to the bathroom or a bright toilet cover, may be helpful. Replacing difficult-to-open zippers and buttons with the Velcro type may help patients to undress. Try to check on them: If you notice that they haven't visited the bathroom for a long time, suggest that they need to do so. Also, watch for clues from body language; remember that AD patients may not always be able to express their needs. Restlessness or a distressed facial expression may sometimes tell you they need to use the bathroom. In the end stages of AD, wearing diapers prevents soaking clothes and bed linen.

84. What can I do if an AD patient wanders?

Unfortunately, wandering is common in patients with moderately advanced AD, and it can happen anytime or at any place. This dangerous behavior raises the risk of patients' being lost, intruding into the wrong places, or being involved in various kinds of accidents. Therefore, it can be life-threatening for them. Because of poor memory and spatial orientation, AD patients can become lost even in familiar settings, and they almost always get lost when they leave the limits of their own neighborhood. Wandering may be triggered by confusion, agitation, and anxiety. It often results from misreading sights and sounds. Some patients who live in the house may have the desire to fulfill former obligations, such as going to work or looking after a child.

By decreasing the number of episodes of confusion and anxiety, you may also decrease the rate of wandering. If episodes of wandering occur, discuss them with your doctor and social worker. Question 75 covers problem behavior and the drug treatment for occasional confusion. The same treatment may reduce the frequency of wandering. You can also limit such wandering by involving patients in productive daily activities, such as cleaning, folding laundry, or preparing dinner. Make sure that patients don't feel lost, abandoned, or disoriented and that they know that they're in the right place. You may also install deadbolt locks on exterior doors, fencing, and gates to prevent AD patients from leaving the limits of their property. Be aware that patients may wander not only by foot but by car, by bus, or by other means. AD patients trying to drive away in a car may create an extremely dangerous situation. For such a possibility, make sure that patients always carry a piece of paper with your name and a phone number where you can be reached. You might also want to enroll that person in the Alzheimer's Association's Safe Return program (discussed in Question 85). You should also keep a list of phone numbers and addresses of the local police, fire departments, and hospitals. If a patient disappears, you should contact the police department and emergency departments of the local hospitals. Many people found wandering on the street are admitted to the hospital for a checkup. Hospital social services and police usually try to contact caregivers, so if a wandering AD patient has a phone number in a pocket, it saves a lot of time and effort.

85. What is "Safe Return"?

Safe Return is a program run by the Alzheimer's Association to assist in the identification and safe, timely return of wandering individuals who have AD and other dementias and have a tendency to become lost. This program is government-funded and has a national range. It started in 1993, and so far about 100,000 individuals have registered. According to Alzheimer's Association statistics, the Safe Return program has a 99% success rate for the safe return of patients registered in the program. Within the last 10 years, 7,500 individuals were recovered and returned to their families and caregivers thanks to Safe Return.

The Safe Return maintains a database containing photos and personal information of registered participants and a 24-hour toll-free emergency crisis line. An AD patient who's enrolled receives identification products that include wallet cards, jewelry, clothing labels, lapel pin, and bag tags. If registered patients wander and are found, the police, emergency medical services, social workers, or private persons may call the toll-free Safe Return number located on patients' identification tags. Safe Return immediately telephones the family or caregivers listed in the database so they can reunite with their loved one. If AD patients are reported missing, the Safe Return database can fax the missing persons' information and photograph to local law enforcement agencies. The Safe Return program also offers behavior education and training for caregivers and families in regard to wandering.

To enroll a patient with dementia, caregivers have to complete an information form containing the patient's name, social security number, height, weight, eye color, distinguishing marks, and other characteristics. Caregivers should enclose the most recent photograph with the application. Caregivers will be asked to provide up to three contact names, addresses, and phone numbers and to choose the type of identification product that the patient will wear or carry. The registration fee is $40. You may register a patient in your local Alzheimer's Association Chapter in person or by phone. Registration forms are available in several languages. You may also register on-line: *https://www.alz. org/resourcecenter/programs/SafeReturnRegister1.asp.* More information about the Safe Return Program is available at *http://www.alz.org/ResourceCenter/Programs/ SafeReturn.htm*

86. What can I do about eating problems (choking, lack of appetite)?

Some patients with advanced dementia may experience less thirst and appetite. This problem may have been going on for a long period and may vary in severity, but it ultimately leads to dehydration and malnutrition. This can be clinically dangerous. Such a situation should prompt medical evaluation to exclude treatable and reversible causes (e.g., constipation, kidney failure, nausea, and fluid and electrolyte imbalance). In some cases, a problem with swallowing is the core of the problem. Many medical conditions may result in affected swallowing and in choking. In such patients, assistance with feeding and drinking can provide some improvement. When you're feeding patients in advanced stages of AD, you have to be sure that they know that they'll be eating. Feeding has to be started slowly and carried out slowly. Surprising or rushing patients may trigger coughing, resistance, and—what may be the worst—aspiration (inhaling food into the lungs). You have to allow about 30 to 40 minutes for each meal. Food and beverages should be either cold or just above room temperature to increase stimulation and to avoid choking.

Unfortunately, some AD patients refuse to drink and eat although they don't suffer from any curable medical problem or swallowing disease. This puts caregivers in an extremely difficult situation. Whether to start artificial food and drink intake in response to a patient's refusal to eat or drink is a difficult question. Because this refusal may be transitory, initial measures may involve replacing fluids with liquid formulas containing a high amount of calories, protein, fibers, and vitamins. In addition, appetite-enhancing drugs can be administered. When such measures fail, families have to decide whether to start intravenous hydration and tube feeding. Tube feeding is performed through a small tube (a PEG), one end of which is placed in the stomach and the other outside through the skin. Placement of such a tube is relatively easy and a standard procedure performed under short-lasting anesthesia. PEG tubes provide an easy, reliable way to give patients nutrients and drugs. Although PEGs are fully reversible and can be removed easily without surgery, families have to realize that prolonging life in this way is in fact lengthening the dying process. Therefore, knowing the patient's point of view on this issue is important. Unfortunately, we can't know that in the end stage of dementia, but you can approach these issues at the beginning of the disease, and patients can formulate their wishes about end-stage care in a living will (discussed in Question 91).

87. Is long-distance caregiving manageable?

Very often, AD patients' closest family members (children or siblings) live beyond commuting distance. This may become a problem when patients require an increased amount of care. Not uncommonly, older adults resist suggestions of moving closer to family members. Many older people don't want to leave the neighborhood where they have lived for many years and where all things are familiar to them. Sometimes, moving closer isn't advisable (e.g., when a family lives in a very hot or very cold climate). An alternative option is for the children to move closer to the patient. However, in many situations, this is even less acceptable, as it requires changing job arrangements. In such situations, so called long-distance care giving may become an alternate option. This can be made to work at an acceptable level, but caring for a loved one who lives far away is often emotionally and financially exhausting.

Distant caregivers are given to guilt and anxiety because they can't personally check on their beloved ones. Some tips and suggestions can help you to make long-distance care giving more manageable and less stressful. First, you should figure out what kind of assistance may be needed. The best way to do that is to spend some time with AD patients who live alone and watch them perform various daily tasks. First, check how they're doing with shopping and cooking. Is there enough of the proper food available in the neighborhood, or does getting it require a ride to a distant supermarket? How are they doing with cooking? Are they eating regular meals? Second, how are they dealing with financial matters? Are they paying the rent, the utilities, and credit cards in time? You should also check on the condition of their house or apartment. Does it require maintenance or repair? Pay attention to the neighborhood. Did it change? Is it still safe? Take a car ride with such patients to see whether they can still drive safely (discussed in Question 68). Pay attention also to patients' personal hygiene, whether they're routinely bathing and grooming (discussed in Question 81). In what condition are their garments? Talk to friends in the neighborhood. Check to see whether they're visiting patients regularly. Inquire whether patients have constant medical care. Talk to their doctors. Check for any issues you should address.

After determining what may be lacking, try to solve possible problems. We always recommend getting as many reliable people as possible involved in supportive care. You may turn for help to friends or more distant family members living nearby. Often, a distant relative who hasn't seen an AD patient for years but lives nearby may be willing to commit a small amount of time to help with care. You should also explore the social services available in the area.

When you talk to a patient's doctor, ask about social workers. A social worker could help you to obtain, and later on supervise, certain services. Community organizations, such as churches, synagogues, neighborhood groups, and volunteer organizations, can also provide some social and companion services. Shopping and cooking frequently are issues. Your choice here involves asking friends or relatives from patients' neighborhoods to shop and supervise meal preparation. You may obtain social service from Meals on Wheels, guaranteeing that at least one warm meal will be delivered daily. Also, you may hire a part-time home health aid. Usually, a combination of more than one gives the best results. You might have to hire a home health aid when patients need supervised grooming and bathing. You can monitor financial matters from a distance. You should obtain power of attorney (discussed in Questions 91 and 92) and authorization for the bank to perform monetary transactions on behalf of patients. You can have copies of bank statements, mortgage payments, or utility bills sent directly to you. Establishing automatic or "easy" payments of these bills is also frequently an option. Although you're separated by a great distance, you should check on such patients often. Call them yourself, but also establish one or several reliable contact persons who can give you additional information. Contact the doctor's office after each follow-up visit. If you have power of attorney (discussed in Question 91) and you are a health care proxy, you may ask for a copy or a doctor's note after each visit. This will enable you to assess patients' condition and medical needs more easily; try to make as many visits as possible.

As you prepare for long-distance caregiving, you have to realize that these measures will not last forever and that, as the disease progresses, long-distance care may not be enough. You have to be prepared that sooner or later a typical AD patient will have to move either to your home or to an assisted-living facility. If you decide to move a patient to your household, you will be taking on certain additional responsibilities. Patients with advanced AD need a lot of care, so either you or another family member will have to devote large amounts of time daily. You have to ask yourself how this arrangement will affect your job, your family, and your finances. You should discuss this idea with the rest of your family and make sure that they support you fully. Check also to see whether social services are available in your area and whether hiring a home health aid makes sense. You should also check to see that your home is equipped and safe for a patient with advanced AD. An important issue is also whether such a patient gives consent to move. Convincing AD patients to move may not be easy and is never achieved with the first try. You should be persistent and slowly build up to the concept of moving. Although it takes time and effort, most patients finally accept the idea of changing their environment. When the patient arrives at your house, you should be aware that moving a person with AD from familiar surroundings may cause increased agitation and confusion. Although this reaction usually passes, it may require prescribing some drugs to ease the concern.

If you can't move a loved one into your home, your next option is to move him or her into an assisted-living facility. Even though such a person is in a long-term care facility, you should maintain ongoing communication with the care staff and friends who visit regularly. Try to work with the managing nurse and physician. Arrange to get frequent updates on the patient's condition and progress. Meet with them when you come to visit the patient.

88. What stage is right for placing an AD patient in a residential care facility?

Unfortunately, the majority of AD patients eventually have to enter an institution. This places great emotional and financial burden on caregivers. The right time for doing this varies greatly from case to case and ranges from the middle stage to the very advanced stage of the disease. It mainly depends on whether caregivers are available and on the family's ability to provide adequate care. Usually, middle-stage AD patients require day-long supervision, whereas end-stage patients require 24-hour care, including feeding and providing drugs. Providing care adequate to the stage of disease includes a skilled work force, technical means, space, and experience. Meeting these challenging demands may not be easy. Many caregivers are busy with their professional careers or live far away and can't spend the required time. Other very important things that may lead to placing patients in a facility is their aggressive, unpredictable behavior (discussed in Question 76) or delusions and paranoia (discussed in Questions 72 and 73). Such disorders don't respond well to treatment at home and require the use of stronger drugs. If you can no longer provide care safely at home, relocation to a residential care facility may be your only realistic option.

89. How do I select the right residential care facility?

This question can be answered in two ways. First, what types of residential care facilities are available? Second, how can you be sure that a selected place will live up to your expectations? The types of residential care facilities depend on the level of care required.

- *Retirement housing*: Retirement housing is a living arrangement focused on the comfort of residents with little or no focus on medical problems, including AD. Generally, this kind of setting provides each resident with an apartment or room that includes cooking facilities or provides food service. No round-the-clock staff is available on site in this type of facility. Retirement housing may be the right setting for patients who are in the early stage of AD but can still care for themselves independently and live alone safely.

- *Assisted-living facilities*: Assisted-living facilities are also called **board-and-care homes**. They fill the gap between independent living and a nursing home. The term **assisted living** is applied to a residence that provides living arrangements and services, such as housekeeping, personal assistance with daily activities (e.g., help with bathing), organized recreational activities, and meal preparation. The staff of assisted-living facilities have basic medical training and are prepared to supervise and help with drugs and to take care of residents during a short-term illness. The arrangements of assisted-living facilities can usually accommodate the needs of patients with mild and moderately advanced AD. We recommend, however, that caregivers inquire about specific services provided by a given facility and the level of functioning required of its residents.

- *Skilled nursing facilities*: Skilled nursing facilities, or nursing homes, are facilities providing 24-hour nursing care to their residents. Nursing homes staffs are trained to deal with such issues as nutrition, care planning, recreation, spirituality, and medical care. Unlike those in a hospital, patients are not covered 24 hours a day by physicians, but physicians from a variety of specialties are usually available several times a week to monitor patients' status and adjust drug doses. Skilled nursing facilities are the best choice for people who need round-the-clock care or are receiving ongoing medical treatment. This would include persons with advanced stages of AD or other types of dementia.

- *Continuum care retirement communities*: Continuum care retirement communities (CCRC) are complex

Board-and-care homes
assisted living facilities.

Assisted-living facilities
residence that provides such living arrangements and services as housekeeping, meal preparation, and assistance with daily activities (e.g., help with bathing).

The arrangements of assisted-living facilities can usually accommodate the needs of patients with mild and moderately advanced AD.

facilities where all the different types of services described are available on one campus. Residents will need, however, to move among buildings to receive a level of care adequate to their medical condition and stage of dementia.

When you're looking for residential care facility, we advise you to contact such organizations as the Alzheimer's Association (*www.alz.org*) or the American Association for Home and Services for Aging (*http://www2.aahsa.org*). They'll provide you with a list of such facilities in your neighborhood and explain what kind of service they provide. They may also help you to determine what kind of service you specifically need. When you want to select a facility, you should visit several places and spend time observing what goes on and how patients are treated there. You should talk with staff working directly with residents to see whether they're competent and content in their jobs. You may ask the staff directly whether they're continually trained on dementia care issues. Ask residents and visitors about their opinion of the facility and staff. See whether the residents look happy, comfortable, relaxed, and involved in activities. You should check whether the environment provides safety and security, promotes residents' independence, and agrees with your own preferences for comfort. In most cases, if you're satisfied with the arrangements of a residential care facility, your beloved one should also feel comfortable.

90. How, as a caregiver, can I deal with my own stress?

Taking care of AD patients is a full-time job that frequently leads to feelings of frustration. In addition, you may feel bitter that instead of receiving support from your spouse, you have to spend so much time and effort on care. Moreover, AD patients may exhibit unpredictable behavior that is a challenge to caregivers. Severe mood swings (discussed in Question 76), combativeness (discussed in Questions 69 and 70), verbal or physical aggression, and wandering (discussed in Questions 84 and 85) can add to your frustration and tension. Perhaps four-fifths of caregivers admit to experiencing high levels of stress, and half experience symptoms of depression. You should understand that your good mental and physical conditions are important for both you and your patients. You shouldn't neglect your own physical, mental, and emotional well-being. You can achieve this by regular rest and exercise, eating well-balanced meals, and regularly visiting a physician for checkups. You should take symptoms of exhaustion, stress, sleeplessness, and changes in appetite seriously because ignoring them can cause your physical and mental health to decline.

Other important signs of caregiver stress are anger; periods of helplessness, despair, and depression; and feelings of frustration with the person for whom they're caring. The first step in dealing with stress is to recognize that it exists; the second is seeking help from others. Caregivers under stress often deny that anything is wrong but at the same time withdraw from social activities, friends, family, and contacts with other persons for whom they care. Family members may pull back, avoiding contacts with both patient and caregiver. You should at some point take the initiative to contact family and friends and explain that while AD has changed your lives in some ways, you value their friendship and support. By increasing contacts with other family members, you may get help with care issues and find somebody with whom you may share your concerns and feelings. You can get further help by contacting other caregivers and support groups for caregivers (discussed in Question 94). These groups are created for the purpose of exchanging ideas and can provide suggestions about how to communicate more easily about caregiver stress. You may also seek solutions for certain problems related to an AD patient's care by becoming more skillful in caregiving techniques. Another helpful hint in reducing your stress is to be realistic about what you can do, giving yourself credit for what you've accomplished, and avoiding feeling guilty if you can't do everything on your own. Be aware also of caregiver depression. Depression is a medical illness, four times more likely to strike those older than age 65, and it's very common among caregivers. Unfortunately, in many cases, depression is unrecognized, and many people do not receive appropriate care and treatment. Some symptoms of depression are a depressed or irritable mood, fatigue, loss of energy, feelings of worthlessness, feelings of excessive guilt, suicidal thinking or attempts, difficulty with thinking or concentrating, problems with sleep (including nightmares and sleeplessness), loss of interest or pleasure in usual activities, and changes in appetite and weight. If four or more of these listed symptoms are present for more than a 2-week period, you should seek professional help and obtain a complete medical evaluation. Depression can be treated very effectively with a variety of methods, under the care of a physician.

LEGAL AND FINANCIAL ISSUES RELATED TO AD

91. What legal matters should AD patients and their families be aware of?

AD patient care is costly and may use up a significant portion of a family's assets. Moreover, patients' capacity for making financial and health-related decisions decreases with time. We recommend, therefore, that you start legal and financial planning as soon as a diagnosis of dementia has been made to ensure financial means for future care. An important legal term for both patient and caregivers is **competency**. In the language of the law, competency is the capacity (or ability) to know and understand information about an issue. As dementia progresses, patients' ability to make certain decisions may be restricted. You also have to understand that patients may not be capable of making certain decisions but still be capable of making others. For example, patients may be capable of deciding whether they want, and agree, to sell a house and move into a nursing home but at the same time may not be able to handle accepting a sell offer for the house because they lack the power to weigh whether the offer is fair. Only a court can decide whether AD patients are competent, whereas a psychiatrist can judge and measure their capacity to make particular decisions. Judging the competency of dementia patients is often an issue for lawyers preparing living wills for them, because they don't want the document to be questioned by interested people who may feel that the assets were not divided up to their advantage.

Competency
legal term for the capacity (or ability) to know and understand information about given issues and make decisions about them (e.g., capacity to understand the fact of selling a house and ability to weigh whether an offer for it is fair).

Power of attorney
legal term for a document in which a patient gives a trusted person legal authority to act on his or her behalf; usually given to manage assets or health-related issues or both.

We always recommend that you prepare certain legal documents as early as possible in the disease. Patients might give a trusted person the **power of attorney**. The term refers to the legal document by which a patient (the "principal") gives legal authority to another person (the "agent") to act on their behalf. Other family members should respect a person appointed as an agent; such a person should be trustworthy, good in managing money, and if possible live close by. There are many reasons why preparing a document of power of attorney is helpful. It enables patients to set specific guidelines as to how they want financial matters to be handled and at what time. In this way, many families have avoided going to court to handle financial matters. You can give somebody power of attorney exclusively for managing your assets or health-related issues. The latter form of power of attorney is also called "health care directive" (discussed in Question 92). Another legal document helping to manage your assets is a "living trust," which lists your assets and appoints either a bank or a trusted individual as your trustee. We also recommend that you prepare a will. In the will, you name those people who will receive your estate at the time of your death and an executor who will carry out the will and manage your estate.

In preparing legal documents or consulting on legal matters about patients with dementia, you may consider contacting an attorney specializing in elder law. This is a special area of law focusing on issues that typically affect older adults. You may find such an attorney through the Alzheimer's Association or the National Academy of Elder Law Attorneys, Inc. The latter (*http://www.naela.com/*) is a nonprofit association that assists lawyers, bar organizations, and others who work with older clients and their families. It provides a wealth of information, including its own quarterly published journal, education, networking, and assistance to those who must deal with the many special issues involved with legal services to the elderly and disabled. Once the documents are prepared, copies have to be left with a caregiver or a trusted family member and an attorney. The name, address, and phone number of the person who receives the power of attorney and a copy of a living will should be put into the medical file in the patient's doctor's office.

92. What are advanced directives?

Advanced directives are legal documents that enable patients to record their preferences for treatment and care, including end-of-life wishes. AD patients, like all other patients, have the legal right to limit or forgo medical or life-sustaining treatment, including the use of mechanical ventilators, cardiopulmonary resuscitation, antibiotics, and artificial nutrition and hydration. You should prepare advance directives after discussing details with family and doctors. Your neurologist or your primary-care physician should suggest preparing advanced directives. One or the other should also provide you with advice about options for future medical care. You shouldn't be pressured to prepare advanced directives, however. Remember that discussion of end-of-life issues should take place while AD patients still are able to make decisions. With advance directives, family and physicians will know patients' wishes and can respectfully follow them.

Advance directives take two common forms: a living will and a durable power of attorney for health care. A living will is a document that states your choices for future medical care decisions. These mainly center on the use of artificial life support systems. As stated, all persons have the legal right to limit or forgo medical or life-sustaining treatment (cardiopulmonary resuscitation, mechanical ventilators, antibiotics, feeding tubes, and artificial hydration). Both patients and family members should understand that withdrawal or refusal of treatment, including management for life-threatening illnesses (e.g., stroke, hemorrhage, or heart attacks), can't be compared to **euthanasia** or assisted suicide. In the presence of untreatable end-stage illness, aggressive medical management may feel like torture to an individual in an unfamiliar environment who is unable to understand the intentions of care providers.

Euthanasia
deliberate shortening of life in patients with terminal diseases (e.g., cancer) and typically performed by administrating a lethal dose of medication.

A durable power of attorney for health care (or health care directive) is a legal document that appoints an agent, usually a trusted family member, vesting in him or her a power to make all decisions regarding health care. These decisions include (but are not limited to) selection of health care providers, consent for medical procedures, choices of medical treatment, and end-of-life decisions. The term *durable* means that the agent can act on patients' behalf after they no longer can make decisions themselves. In other words, a person with a durable power of attorney becomes a patient's health care proxy.

93. What are potential sources of coverage for AD-related medical spending?

The truth is that AD is one of the most costly diseases. The financial burden of caring for the 4 million AD patients in the United States is nearly $100 billion a year. Also true is that neither governmental nor most private health insurance covers much of the long-term costs for AD patients. About three-fourths of those with AD live at home with care provided by family and friends. Patients' families pay most of the cost of home-based care, including nursing aids. Private resources also pay most of nursing home care costs, which on average are around $40,000 per year but may be as high as $60,000 to $80,000 yearly. In Question 91, we stressed the importance of financial planning to meet the needs of AD patients. You have to realize the great magnitude of these expenses. You should, however, be aware of various government-provided benefits to help with your spending. U.S. citizens who are 65 years old or older are eligible for Social Security retirement benefits. These include Medicare, which is a federal health insurance program. Information about Medicare can be obtained from its Web site (*http://www.medicare.gov*) or by calling 1-800-772-1213 or 1-800-677-1116. Medicare covers inpatient hospital care, an ample portion of patient's doctor's fees, part of their medication costs, and such other medical expenses as physical and occupational therapies and home health care. These include some (but not all) of the services that AD patients may require. Your local Social Security office processes applications for Medicare. You may obtain coverage for copayments and deductibles required by Medicare by buying Medigap, which is a form of private supplementary insurance. The more expensive policies may cover remaining costs of prescription drugs. The following link from the Medicare's Web site (*http://www.medicare.gov/MGcompare/home.asp)* helps you to find choices of private agencies offering Medigap in your area. You may select one that best fits your financial needs.

Another choice is enrollment in a Medicare HMO (Medicare managed care), which is a medical plan under Medicare. A Medicare HMO offers AD patients an expanded range of benefits, including nursing home and home health care but for limited periods and only under special circumstances. This expansion of benefits is provided in exchange for a limit on patients' choices of hospitals, doctors, and other professionals. This program will basically provide them with a roster of names and places that will limit your choice.

You should also be aware that you can purchase for them a private insurance plan and use it instead of the Medicare/Medigap combination or Medicare HMO. If they're preparing for retirement, in many cases an insurance plan that has been provided by their employer offers continuity of coverage at the rate paid by the employer.

As you probably realize by now, AD patients are expected to cover a portion of the bill for their current medical needs. When you plan for necessary spending in their future, you naturally want to protect your and their assets. Ideally, you should begin financial planning soon after a diagnosis of dementia has been made. Retirement benefits should provide a bulk of critical financial resources. These may include retirement plans, individual retirement accounts (IRAs), annuities, Social Security, and investment assets (stocks and bonds, savings accounts, real estate, etc.). You must also remember that Medicare does not cover the costs of nursing homes or home health aid. You have to cover these expenses directly out of pocket. If resources from their retirement benefits were exhausted, you'd have to look for other sources of income, such as personal property (jewelry and artwork) or real estate. You can take out for them either a home equity loan or a reverse mortgage on a home. Another option is to sell real estate and invest the money to cover their cost of nursing home care.

The government provides social support for those who have minimal income, cash, or other assets. Medicaid is a federal program that may cover costs of long-term care of those AD patients with limited financial resources. Although Medicaid is a federal program, typically each state's welfare agency administers it, with the result that eligibility and benefits vary from state to state. Depending on individual circumstances, Medicaid can cover all or a portion of nursing home costs. You may obtain more information by visiting the Health Care Financing Administration (HCFA) Web site: *http://www.hhs.gov/medicaid.*

Medicaid is a federal program that may cover costs of long-term care of those AD patients with limited financial resources.

Social Security disability is a program to assist those wage earners who are younger than age 65 and can no longer work because they're disabled. Applicants must have worked a minimum of 5 nonconsecutive years in the last 10 years and must establish their disability status. In this case, AD or some other form of illness is the reason for disability. You should submit a physician's statement with a description of the diagnosis, the extent of disability, and other medical documentation of the disease to your local Social Security office. Information is available at the Social Security Administration's Web site: *http://www.ssa.gov.*

Those AD patients who are aged 65 or over and have limited income and assets can enroll in the supplemental security income program that guarantees a minimum monthly income to disabled persons.

Some nonprofit organizations may also provide financial resources for people with limited assets. You may contact the Alzheimer's Family Relief Program in the American Health Assistance Foundation by calling 1-800-437-2423, or you can visit their Web page: *http://www.ahaf.org/afrp/app.htm.*

94. How can I obtain help for managing an AD patient at home?

Taking care of an AD patient is a full-time occupation. Many caregivers may not be able to meet such a time commitment. Additionally, many caregivers who can commit the required amount of time to patient care may also require some help as they become tired and stressed. In both cases, they'll require some form of external support. Home health care services may provide health care assistance to AD patients in their homes. As a first step, a given agency conducts an assessment of the needs of an AD patient. Then the agency works with a doctor to develop a plan of care. Sometimes the doctor is the one who prompts the agency providing health care assistance directly. Home health care service employees are medically trained and provide a broad spectrum of services (e.g., assisting with giving drugs, changing dressings, or checking blood pressure). You can obtain help from your doctor in finding an agency providing home health care service. Then, too, you can contact government agencies, such as the Administration on Aging (*http://www.aoa.dhhs.gov*), or private organizations, such as the Alzheimer's Association (*http://www.alz.org*).

Another form of home-based support for caregivers is respite care, mainly offered through community organizations or residential facilities. This form of service may provide temporary relief from the tasks of care-giving. Their help may include companion services, personal care, household assistance, and skilled care services to meet specific patient needs. You can employ in-home helpers privately through an agency or as part of a government program. Also, adult day services may provide opportunities to interact with other patients or people in a community center or facility.

PART FIVE

Searching for the Cure

Are any new therapeutic and diagnostic
approaches under development?

Can AD-damaged nerve cells be restored?

What are the pros and cons of joining
a clinical trial? How do I join?

More ...

95. Are any new therapeutic and diagnostic approaches under development?

AD is among the most intensively studied illnesses in medical science nowadays. The federal government alone spent nearly $600 million on AD-related research in the year 2002. Although the total research spending pool—after adding funds provided by private, nonprofit organizations, and by biotech and pharmaceutical companies—is much higher, this still represents a minute portion of the $100 billion spent annually to cover the cost of care for 4 million AD patients. Thanks to money devoted to research and development, scientists are trying to understand the mechanism of the disease better, to produce better animal models, and to develop new diagnostic and therapeutic approaches. Many clinical trials are under way, focused on slowing AD's progression. These trials include testing of cholesterol-lowering agents, hormones, Ginkgo, and anti-inflammatory and antioxidant drugs (discussed in the Treatment section). Although we have reasons to hope that some of these tested agents may retard the advance of disease, they're not primarily targeting AD. We understand well that the greatest success can be achieved only by halting or reversing the underlying mechanism of AD. Many research laboratories target **amyloidosis-β** as their treatment focus. Scientists have proposed a number of approaches against the buildup and deposit of amyloid-β, and many of them are successful in treating amyloid-β deposits in AD transgenic mice models. These include a new, safer generation of vaccine compounds that can bind to amyloid-β and eliminate it from the blood, preventing deposits in the brain. Others are compounds called "β-**sheet breakers**," which can enter

Amyloidosis-β
process of depositing of amyloid-β in the brain in AD.

β-Sheet breakers
compounds designed to bind to amyloid-β and prevent formation of amyloid-β plaques.

the brain and slow amyloid-β buildup. Other compounds are designed to neutralize the bad effect of apolipoprotein E, the presence of which increases buildup of amyloid-β deposits. Last, scientists are trying to develop compounds inhibiting β and γ secretases (β and γ secretases), which are enzymes responsible for the production of amyloid-β. These agents are called β and γ **secretase inhibitors**. Some of these approaches are entering the initial phases of human clinical trials.

As mentioned, no exact diagnostic test for AD exists. We also believe that amyloid-β accumulates in the brain for years before the clinical onset of dementia symptoms. Therefore, many laboratories are trying to develop methods that would directly show amyloid-β plaques. Such a method would allow us to identify persons at risk, before irreversible damage to their nerve cells occurs, and to chart the effectiveness of therapy against amyloid-β.

Three approaches are under development, and so far they have succeeded in detecting plaques in AD transgenic mice. The first approach uses special compounds to bind to amyloid plaques and change the signal detected by magnetic resonance imaging (MRI). The second approach uses MRI with a particularly strong magnetic field to show plaques directly. The third concept is based on using compounds labeled with an isotope; they bind to plaques and can be recognized by a positron emission tomography (PET) scanner. The last approach has entered initial clinical trials in humans.

If you're interested in financially supporting research about AD, you can obtain helpful information from your local Alzheimer's Disease Association chapter

Secretase inhibitors line of experimental drugs for AD currently under development and designed to inhibit function of β- or γ-secretases and thereby decrease the amount of amyloid-β produced.

Searching for the Cure

(*www.alz.org*) or by contacting your nearest Alzheimer's Disease Research Center (listed with links at *http://www.alzheimers.org/adcdir.htm*).

96. Can AD-damaged nerve cells be restored?

Some cells in the body (skin, for example) can divide and replace those that have died or have been damaged. Unfortunately, mature nerve cells have a very limited ability to regenerate, and the majority can't divide. They make up for losses by making denser connections between existing cells. Although upcoming new treatment approaches for AD carry a promise to halt the disease process, these treatments can't rebuild what's already destroyed. The same remains true for many other neurodegenerative diseases. Different approaches are being developed to help the mature brain to regenerate nerve cells. These approaches use so-called **stem cells** from bone marrow. Stem cells can be made to divide and turn into adult nerve cells. Laboratory experiments in animal models have shown that certain stem cells can be transplanted into the brain and will grow and function as normal brain cells. This research is still in the early stages, although it has shown some very promising results. Scientists continue to learn more about how stem cells grow and how they become different types of body cells, including the various cell types found in the brain. If they can find a way to control these cells and direct them to damaged areas of the brain, it would lead to new treatments not only for AD but for stroke, Parkinson's disease, and other neurodegenerative disorders.

Another research approach that scientists are seriously pursuing is injecting **neurotrophic growth factors**.

Stem cells

cells in the bone marrow that have the capacity of turning into other cells of the body.

Neurotrophic growth factors

substances that can stimulate nerve cells to grow their processes over long distances and form new connections with other nerve cells.

Neurotrophic growth factors are substances that stimulate nerve cells to grow their processes over long distances and form new connections with other nerve cells. They are absolutely necessary for normal brain growth and development that occurs during the fetal period and in infants. Later on, during adult life, their levels in the brain decrease. Researchers are studying whether introducing neurotrophic growth factors in dementia patients may start regeneration and halt cognitive decline. A major problem with the use of this compound is that in their natural form, neurotrophic growth factors don't enter the brain if injected into the bloodstream or given in pill form. To overcome this obstacle, scientists have developed such drugs as Propentofylline or Neotrofin, which can be given by mouth and have the properties of growth factors. Small clinical trials have demonstrated that AD patients who received these drugs have clinically measurable decrease in dementia symptoms, whereas those patients who received placebo (dummy drugs) got worse. Similar results have been shown for vascular dementia.

Another tested method of delivery of growth factors into the brain uses gene therapy. Genetically altered tissue capable of producing growth factors would be surgically implanted into a patient's brain. The first such implant was performed at the University of California San Diego School of Medicine in April 2001 in a 60-year-old woman in the early stage of AD. This preliminary study was designed to study whether the gene transplantation was safe. After having proved that, researchers will launch a larger study to weigh the effectiveness of this kind of treatment.

97. How are new therapies introduced into clinical practice?

The current extensive research on AD has generated and will continue to generate bright ideas that can be turned into new treatment approaches. Scientists first test both the effectiveness and the potentially harmful effect of these approaches in the test tube and on animals. If these studies produce promising results, doctors/researchers will start clinical trials on humans. Remember that clinical trials are performed by U.S. licensed physicians who specialize in treating AD and in conducting clinical investigations as well. All new drug trials are being approved and supervised by the U.S. Food and Drug Administration. This governmental agency is responsible for approving all new drugs for clinical use. This agency has two major concerns: Are new drugs really effective in treating disease symptoms, and are the new drugs are safe? Proof of drug effectiveness and lack of toxicity is required for registering new drugs. This information is gathered through three phases of clinical trials. Phase I clinical trials experiment on a small group of volunteers, and they focus mainly on the safety of a new drug. Results of phase I trials can already shed some light on a drug's effectiveness. Phase II clinical trials usually involve several hundreds of volunteers and serve multiple purposes, including further safety monitoring, recording the rate of side effects, establishing the right dosage, and studying the treatment effect. Phase III clinical trials test thousands of patients using experience gathered from the phase II trials of side effects and dosages. They seek to extend the experience from possible side effects of a drug and weigh its effect on disease symptoms in a large population. Many phase I trials and small phase II trials take place at a single

The current extensive research on AD has generated bright ideas that can be turned into new treatment approaches.

site, especially at locations near Bethesda, MD, the home of the U.S. National Institutes of Health (NIH). Larger phase II and phase III trials often occur at multiple sites across the United States.

This method of introducing drugs into clinical practice is complex but makes sense. For example, phase I trials offered no evidence about the toxicity of the AD vaccine from animal models. During the phase II trial, doctors saw toxic effects in 6% of vaccinated subjects within the first year of treatment. This stopped the trial, although overall most vaccinated patients showed some lessening of their dementia. Many promising new drugs are under development, and many patients and caregivers are tempted to try them. However, until clinical trials are finished, we don't know the true usefulness and safety of these drugs. What was effective and safe for mice doesn't have to be effective and safe for humans. So, until clinical testing is fully performed, offering these drugs to patients is illegal. Patients may join a clinical trial to help in these research efforts.

98. What are the pros and cons of joining a clinical trial? How do I join?

Clinical trials are designed to introduce to clinical practice drugs that scientists and doctors hope will improve the outcome of a disease. As described, clinical trials take place in different stages. Usually, investigating physicians organize large recruitments for phases II and III. The biggest benefit from joining a clinical trial is starting a novel drug before it becomes available on the market. Previous experiences demonstrate that many drugs tested in clinical trials later become very successful in treating many diseases. In this way, trials have proved the efficacy of cholinesterase inhibitors (discussed in Questions 52–55) and memantine (discussed in Question 56) on improving memory test scores of AD patients. Two kinds of clinical trials are offered to AD patients. One type tests a drug already FDA-approved for a disorder different from AD. Doctors start these trials either because of laboratory data or because of accidental clinical observations. Examples of this are trials of nonsteroidal inflammatory agents (discussed in Question 51) and cholesterol-lowering drugs—statins (discussed in Question 59)—to treat AD. In both situations, direct evidence from laboratory studies and disease statistics showed that these drugs may slow down the AD process. So, testers used them directly in clinical trials to confirm this idea. The clinical trials of anti-inflammatory agents so far have not shown their benefit. The clinical trial testing statins as a treatment for AD is ongoing, and the physicians directing the trial are very optimistic. In this type of trial, they know potential risks and side effects of the drugs from previous use.

In the second type of situation, investigating doctors introduce a completely new drug to clinical trials on the basis of the strength of laboratory evidence that it may target some crucial mechanism. In this type of study, doctors have limited evidence about potentially harmful effects. This evidence comes from testing the drug on animals. They assume that the drug is free of potential side effects, but this must be tested during the trial. Obviously, U.S.-licensed physicians wouldn't risk patients' health if they knew that a new drug could be dangerous.

If you're interested in enrolling in a study, take the following information into consideration. As has been emphasized, you'd have to understand that clinical studies seek to find out the effectiveness and safety of a drug. Volunteering may involve some risk, since the treatments being tested are still considered experimental. Remember also that if physicians discover some adverse affects, they'll notify the volunteers, and the study will be stopped. Another thing you have to realize is that not all participants are given the medication being tested. In almost all studies, participants are divided into two groups: an experimental group (those members receive the active drug) and a control group (those members receive a placebo, also called a dummy drug or "sugar pill"). Neither participants nor investigating drug physicians know who's taking the active drug and who's in the placebo group. A third party involved in collecting data for the study records this information and releases it to the investigators and participants once the study is completed. This type of study design provides unbiased testing of a drug's usefulness. If, during the study, a drug demonstrates a significant effect, doctors immediately offer the true drug to those patients taking the sugar pills.

If you enroll in a clinical trial, you or your caregiver may have to answer questions about your condition. After you contact a study center, your first conversation with investigating physicians usually includes a phone interview to find out whether you're suited for the study. Questions may include "When was a diagnosis of Alzheimer's made? Are you are in generally good health? and Do you reside at home or in a facility?" The investigators will also want to know whether a caregiver can be available to assist you during the study. The next step would involve comprehensive medical testing, including general medical and nervous system examinations; imaging studies, such as computed tomography (CT) or magnetic resonance imaging (MRI); and blood and urine tests. These studies will help to decide whether you're a suitable candidate and, if you are, the extent of your deficit caused by AD at the moment the trial begins. These tests and routine follow-up examinations are free of charge to you.

If you want to be involved in a study, you have to be aware of the commitment and responsibilities required from both patients and caregivers. Researchers conducting the study rely on caregivers to administer a drug according to schedule, return with the patient to the study site for regular follow-up visits, and report any changes in the patient's condition or behavior. In so many ways, caregivers are just as involved as patients are in the study, because AD patients may not be able to identify problems, such as constipation and drowsiness, that may result from the use of drugs. During enrollment, you shouldn't be afraid to ask questions about the study. You or your caregiver can inquire about possible side effects of the test drug, potential benefits, schedule of receiving the drug, and time commitment related to follow-up visits. The researcher should be able to answer any questions you may have throughout the study. If you're not satisfied with the answers at any time, you may be best served to discontinue the study. Not everyone will be willing or qualified to become a research participant. However, those who do participate have the satisfaction of being involved in the development of a potential treatment of AD. You can obtain information about ongoing clinical trials from the Alzheimer's Association (*http://www.alz.org/ResourceCenter/ByTopic/ClinicalTrials.htm*) or from the National Institutes of Health (*www.clinicaltrials.gov*). You can learn which trials are ongoing and which are recruiting and whom to contact for recruitment.

99. Should AD patients and their families agree to donate the patient's brain for research after death?

Many physicians involved in the care of AD patients are also involved in research on this disease. Studies on human tissue can lead to better understanding of the origin of the disease and how it progresses. Even the best animal models can't replace human tissue in this respect. Larger medical centers specializing in AD programs have laboratories where scientists are studying human tissue. The availability of human brains for AD research is critical. Patients receiving care in specialized clinical centers are well known to the personnel, and clinical histories of their disease are well documented. Therefore, a request for organ donation after patients' death is frequent and should not be surprising. Usually, when a family receives such a request, they're given reading material describing the process of organ donation and an opportunity to ask questions freely. AD patients, or their health care proxies, can agree on donation at any time and can change their minds at any time. If they believe that donation may interfere with religious beliefs or practice, they are advised to contact a clergy member to discuss this issue. Representatives from different faiths are available in a medical center through the pastoral care service. In the event of death, the autopsy is provided free of charge and performed in a way that does not interfere with funeral arrangements. The autopsy may be limited only to removal of the brain (which does not leave marks visible on the body and does not interfere with an open-casket funeral). The family has the right to learn the results of the autopsy and how the brain is going to be used for research.

100. Where can I find more information?

As a patient, caregiver, or family member, you may have specific questions or want to contact other caregivers or specialists. The Appendix that follows offers resources.

Organizations

Alzheimer's Association
225 North Michigan Avenue
Suite 1700
Chicago, Illinois 60601-7633
Pjone: 800-272-3900; 312-335-8700
Fax: 312-335-1110
www.alz.org

American Health Assistance Foundation
22512 Gateway Center Drive,
Clarksburg, Maryland 20871
1-800-437-2423, (301) 948-3244,
Fax: (301) 258-9454
www.ahaf.com

National Institute on Aging
Alzheimer's Disease Education and Referral Center
1-800-438-4380
http://www.alzheimers.org/index.html

National Institutes of Health
Information about clinical trials
www.clinicaltrials.gov

Clinical Trials

http://www.alz.org/ResourceCenter/ByTopic/ClinicalTrials.htm
Web pages updated by these organizations also offer an opportunity to ask specific questions and list questions and answers asked by caregivers and patients. You can also ask questions by calling listed 1-800 numbers of organizations' hotlines for patients and caregivers.

By contacting them, you may obtain information about:

- Recent advances in the field of Alzheimer's disease
- Tips on care giving
- Meetings of caregivers groups
- How to find a specialist in your area
- How to obtain social help
- Clinical trials

To increase your knowledge about AD, you may also want to explore other Web pages devoted to education on AD:
The National Institute of Health Alzheimer's Disease General Information web site:
http://www.alzheimers.org/generalinfo.htm

Jenssen Pharmaceutical Inc.
http://www.gcrweb.com/alzheimersDSS/

NeuroCAST (an educational program of Athena Diagnostics)
http://www.neurocast.com/site/content/sessions_archived.asp

Physicians for AD Patients

- Explore *U.S. News & World Report's* yearly published list of the top 50 medical centers in each specialty at:
  http://www.usnews.com/usnews/nycu/health/hosptl/rankings/specihqneur.htm,
- Obtain information from Alzheimer's Disease Association chapters. See Alzheimer's Disease Association contact listed above.
- Browse Web page or a directory of a medical center near you. Look for specific terms (e.g., dementia, Alzheimer's disease, memory clinic, or center for brain health).

Medical Coverage for AD Patients

Every U.S. citizen who is 65 years old or older is entitled to governmental health benefits distributed through Medicare.

To contact Medicare services
http://www.medicare.gov
1-800-772-1213 or 1-800-677-1116.

Supplemental medicare insurance (Medigap) can be obtained through many private insurance companies. Search of such company operating in your neighbourhood can be performed through following a Medicare-approved Web page: *http://www.medicare.gov/MGcompare/home.asp*

Miscellaneous

Safe Return (Program of Alzheimer's Association to find AD patients with a tendency to wander and get lost):

Information: *http://www.alz.org/ResourceCenter/Programs/SafeReturn.htm*

Registration: *https://www.alz.org/resourcecenter/programs/SafeReturnRegister1.asp.*

or by phone (see above).

Medicolegal issues

You may find an attorney who specializes in legal issues arising in aged individuals (e.g., preparation of living will, power of attorney, trust funds or other documents).

These lawyers are associated with the Alzheimer's Association or the National Academy of Elder Law Attorneys, Inc. You may contact the National Academy of Elder Law Attorneys on their Web page *http://www.naela.com/*

Residential Care Facilities

A list of facilities by location is available at the Alzheimer's Association site (*www.alz.org*) or American Association for Home and Services for Aging (*http://www2.aahsa.org*).

Glossary

α-synuclein: Protein that builds up in excessive amounts in nerve cells in Parkinson's disease and Lewy-body dementia. Accumulation of α-synuclein in nerve cells causes Lewy bodies. Accumulation of α-synuclein in nerve cells leads to their dysfunction and death.

Abstract thinking: Thinking about imaginary ideas and symbolic meaning of things

Acetylcholine: An activating neurotransmitter indispensable for the brain's cognitive process

AD: Alzheimer's disease.

AD transgenic animals: Genetically altered animals, usually mice, that are designed to mimic AD. These animals do not develop AD exactly as humans do, but they show certain aspects of disease (e.g., amyloid-β plaques or neurofibrillary tangles. They are used to develop new drugs and diagnostic tests.

Allele: A copy of a gene. Most of genes have two copies, therefore two alleles. In certain genetic diseases, alteration (mutation) of both alleles is required for symptoms to appear; in others, such as genetically determined young-onset AD, mutation of only one allele leads to occurrence of the disease.

Ambulatory: Able to walk.

Amino acid: A single chemical compound used by nature to build proteins.

Amygdala: Part of the brain associated with feeling emotions.

Amyloid precursor protein: A large protein that includes amyloid-β. In healthy people, excess of amyloid precursor protein is destroyed so that it does not cause increased amyloid-β. In AD, amyloid precursor protein is destroyed in a manner associated with release of excess of amyloid-β. Enzymes that cut out amyloid-β from the amyloid precursor protein are called β- and γ-secretases.

Amyloid-β: Abnormal protein derived from a larger protein (the amyloid precursor protein) that is deposited in the brain in AD.

Amyloidosis-β: Process of depositing of amyloid-β in the brain in AD. Amyloidosis-β is associated with neuronal loss and dementia. Therefore, preventing or slowing this process is currently an intense area of research leading to development of a cure for AD.

Anorexia: Severe and prolonged lack of apetite leading to significant loss of weight and malnutrition. This condition can be life-threatening.

Antibody: Specific protein that is produced by the immune system and can neutralize and destroy infectious agents (e.g., bacteria or viruses).

Anticonvulsant: Medication given to stop or prevent seizures.

Antiemetic: Medication given to stop or prevent nausea and vomiting.

Antioxidant: Compound capable of neutralizing free radicals. Vitamin E is an example.

Antipsychotic medications: Class of medication used to treat psychosis, delusions, and agitation in AD patients

Anxiolytics: Class of medication used to treat anxiety and agitation

Aphasia: Inability to speak, write, or understand language

Apolipoprotein E: Protein transporting cholesterol in the brain and in the blood. It exists in three forms—E2, E3, E4—in various peo-ple. These born with the E4 form are at increased risk for AD.

Apraxia: Inability to perform certain tasks (e.g., cutting bread, waving good-bye) despite preservation of strength. The problem is usually associated with a neurodegenerative disease and related to losing ability to execute once-learned tasks.

Aspartame: An amino acid that is a natural element found in many food products Because it tastes sweet but has no calories, it is often used as a sugar substitute. (See also phenylalanine).

Aspiration pneumonia: Form of pneumonia caused by aspiration of food into the lungs. It may occur in persons who have difficulties with swallowing. This condition is very serious and requires treatment with intravenous antibiotics.

Assisted-living facilities: Residence that provides living arrangements and services such as housekeeping, meal preparation, and assistance with daily activities (e.g., help with bathing). Frequently, assisted-living facilities also organize recreational activities. (See question 89.)

Atherosclerosis: Deposits of cholesterol in walls of arteries, resulting in their hardening and narrowing; predisposes to strokes (in case of process involving brain arteries) or heart attack (when heart arteries are involved)

Atrophy: Shrinkage, loss of volume; here used in contexts of atrophy of the brain and loss of brain volume

Audiogram: A test to evaluate hearing.

Automatic implanted cardiac defibrillator: Device implanted into a patient's chest that is able to detect life-threatening abnormalities of cardiac rhythm and automatically deliver small electric shocks to bring heart rhythm back to normal. Because such cardiac defibrillators can be triggered by a magnetic field, people in whom it was installed must not undergo magnetic resonance imaging.

Autosomal dominant: The way in which genetic diseases are inherited. Genes usually exist in pairs, called alleles. In autosomal dominant genetic diseases, passing only one mutated allele (gene copy) is sufficient to produce disease in the next generation. In contrast, autosomal recessive diseases occur only if two alleles (gene copies) are affected. All known inherited forms of AD are transmitted in autosomal dominant fashion. One affected allele causes symptoms of disease.

β-Sheet breakers: Compounds designed to bind to amyloid-β and prevent formation of amyloid-β plaques. Effectiveness of these compounds has been shown in transgenic AD mouse models.

Basal ganglia: Structures deep in the brain (*see also* **gray matter**) responsible for making movement smooth and precise. They are damaged in Parkinson's disease, which is associated with shaking of the hands, impaired walking, and falls.

Beta blockers: Heart medications used to slow heart rate and lower blood pressure.

Binswanger's disease: Form of vascular dementia caused by closing off small vessels supplying the white matter of the brain. Damage to these small vessels occurs as a result of uncontrolled elevated blood pressure and diabetes.

Biological reserve: Surplus of capacity of a given organ or system in the body; has to be destroyed before symptoms of the disease occur. For example, studies have shown that initial problems with learning and memory appear in AD after almost 50% of nerve cells in certain parts of the hippocampus are gone.

Blood-brain barrier: Tight layer surrounding blood vessels running through the brain. The blood-brain barrier prevents certain toxins from getting into the brain from the blood stream. Conversely, such toxic substances as amyloid-β are actively removed from the brain by active transport through the blood-brain barrier. Dysfunction of the blood-brain barrier in sporadic AD results in impaired removal of amyloid-β from the brain and allows amyloid-β from the bloodstream to enter the brain. This leads to accumulation of amyloid-β in the brain.

Board-and-care homes: Also called assisted living facilities.

Brain cortex: Superficial layer of the brain composed of nerve cells. Most intellectual functions (e.g., language, graphic, mathematical skills, judgment) are located in specific parts of the cortex. Cortex is also a place for long-term information storage (long-term memory).

Capgrass syndrome: Belief by a person with advanced dementia that relatives are imposters.

Cardiac arrhythmia: Heart rate abnormality

Cardiopulmonary bypass machine: Device designed to replace function of the heart temporarily (pumping of the blood) and the lungs (oxygenation of the blood); used during complicated heart surgeries (when the heart has to be stopped). Its use is associated with increased risk of stroke

Cardiovascular disease: Disease affecting heart (e.g., coronary artery disease and heart failure) and large arteries leading to their occlusion; in turn may result in a stroke or painful ulceration in calves or feet (when a leg artery becomes occluded). Elevated blood pressure, elevated cholesterol, diabetes, and smoking are common risk factors for cardiovascular diseases.

Cardiovascular system: Heart and blood vessels.

Cerebrospinal fluid: Fluid surrounding and cushioning the brain. It becomes altered in various brain diseases; therefore, investigation of cerebrospinal fluid may give a physician clues to diagnosis. A sample of cerebrospinal fluid is obtained during a procedure called spinal tap.

Cholinesterase inhibitors: Class of medications used to improve and slow symptoms of AD dementia by increasing the amount of acetylcholine in the brain. Their use is currently a standard of care for AD patients.

Chromosome: Structure carrying DNA-encoding proteins. Humans have 23 pairs of chromosomes.

Chronic obstructive pulmonary disease: Prolonged bronchitis resulting from many years of smoking or exposure to toxic fumes. Symptoms include shortness of breath, gasping, and decreased exercise tolerance. Patients with this disorder are prone to develop spasms of bronchi and infection that may worsen this condition.

Cisternogram: Study performed to investigate whether a patient with normal-pressure hydrocephalus would be a good candidate for a shunting procedure. During this test, a small amount of radioisotope is injected into the cerebrospinal fluid, and physicians using a special camera may determine signs of cerebrospinal fluid flow blockage.

Cognition: Unique ability of the human brain allowing us to explore the world. Cognition involves many aspects such as abstract thinking, judgment, language, memory, learning, mathematical, and graphic (visuospatial) skills.

Cognitive process: Process of exploring the world thanks to multiple abilities of human brain.

Competency: Legal term for the capacity or ability to know and understand information about given issues and make decision about them (e.g., capacity to understand the fact of selling a house and ability to weigh whether an offer for it is fair). Competency in AD patients is usually limited and decreases as the disease progresses. Only a court can decide whether an AD patient is competent, whereas a psychiatrist can judge and measure a patient's ability to make particular decisions.

Complex partial seizure: Form of seizures associated with impaired consciousness.

Consolidation of memory: Technical term describing structural changes that take place in the hippocampus during learning and allow us to learn and remember things.

Coronary artery disease: Narrowing of heart arteries by deposits of cholesterol in their walls (atherosclerosis). This condition can lead to heart attacks.

Corticobasal ganglionic degeneration: Rare form of neurodegenerative disease leading to dementia and motor dysfunction.

Dehydration: Medical term describing condition in which a patient's system is deficient in water. Patients reaching the severe stage of this condition may be unable to maintain adequate blood pressure and have decreased production of urine, and some AD patients may even experience worsening of dementia. Dehydration is caused either by inadequate water consumption or huge losses of water (e.g., excessive urination). It is treated by replacement of fluids, which may be performed intravenously in severe cases.

Delirium: Acute change in mental status associated with irrational behavior and agitation. Delirium is a medical emergency requiring evaluation in an emergency department.

Delusions: False beliefs not shared by others. They tend to be maintained firmly even if they don't agree with reality and even if they are strongly contradicted by others. Examples of delusions typically associated with AD are delusions of infidelity (belief in an unfaithful spouse) or delusions of theft (belief that valuables are being stolen).

Dementia: Progressive reduction in multiple intellectual skills, such as memory, language, judgment, and problem solving and resulting from acquired disease of the brain such as AD.

Diabetes: Disease associated with chronically elevated blood sugar level leading to damage of small vessels in kidneys, eyes, and brain, and causing atherosclerosis in large arteries feeding the brain and heart. It may result in strokes or heart attacks, respectively. There are two types of diabetes. Type I occurs in teenagers and is a result of destruction of pancreatic cells producing insulin, a hormone causing cells to consume glucose. This type requires life-long supplementation of insulin. Type II occurs in people between 45 and 60 years of age and is associated with obesity. In type II diabetes, insulin is present, but its action is not sufficient to bring the sugar level down to normal. Type II is treated with oral agents and with insulin as an adjunct therapy. Both types I and II of diabetes increase risk for damage of small and large arteries.

Diuretics: Medications used to increase urine output and used to treat hypertension and heart and kidney failure

Electroencephalogram: Recording of electrical activity of the brain, used to detect and characterize seizures

Electrolytes: General name for a number of ions (e.g., sodium, calcium, potassium, and others) that have to be maintained at an appropriate level in the serum. Disturbances in serum levels of certain metabolites (electrolyte imbalance) may cause seizures or a change in mental status.

Embolus: Blood clot or other material (e.g., fat) that travels with the bloodstream and can lodge in an artery too small to allow it to pass. An embolus lodging in the brain artery may cause a stroke.

Encephalitis: Brain inflammation

Enzyme: Protein facilitating a chemical reaction in the body (e.g., cutting other proteins in half). An example would be γ-secretase, which cuts the amyloid precursor protein, liberating amyloid-β.

Epidemiological studies: Studies aiming to determine frequency of given diseases in the population and their association with such factors as age and gender or with other diseases (e.g., diabetes, elevated cholesterol, or cancer). Epidemiological studies have shown a strong association between AD and advancing age, but there is no such association between AD and gender. Similarly, epidemiological studies have proved an increased risk for AD in people with elevated cholesterol and diabetes, but no association between AD and, say, cancer has been detected.

Erotomania: Excessive interest and preoccupation with sexual matters that may be associated with AD or other forms of dementia as a result of destroying parts of the brain responsible for controlling and suppressing urges and impulses

Estrogen: Female sexual hormone

Euthanasia: Deliberate shortening of life in patients with terminal diseases (e.g., cancer) and typically performed by administrating a lethal dose of medication

Extrapyramidal symptoms: Group of symptoms, including stiffening of the body, involuntary movements, restlessness (a constant need to pace or to fuss with objects), and tremor. They can be associated with Parkinson's disease, Huntington's chorea, or the use of some antipsychotic drugs.

Familial disease: Disease caused by a genetic inherited defect and running in families. Familial disease may affect all members of a given family or only some, but usually more than one person is affected.

Focal seizures: Form of seizures associated with uncontrollable shaking of one limb or half of the body while a patient usually remains conscious

Food and Drug Administration (FDA): Federal government agency in charge of controlling food toxicity and approving medications entering the U.S. pharmaceutical market.

Free radicals: Toxic metabolites of various chemical reactions taking place in the body. Inability to neutralize free radicals successfully is considered a reason for nerve death in certain neurodegenerative diseases (e.g., Parkinson's disease and, to a lesser extent, AD).

Frontotemporal dementia: Neurodegenerative disease much rarer than AD and also leading to dementia; the course of disease is dominated by loss of social inhibition, impaired judgment, and abstract thinking as opposed to impaired memory characteristic of AD.

Gastritis: Inflammation of the stomach

Gastrointestinal surgery: Surgery performed on the gastrointestinal (alimentary) system

Gene: Fragment of DNA coding specific proteins. Most human genes exist as pairs.

Gene mutation: Defect in a gene that alters the protein it codes, usually causing a disease. Gene mutations can either be inherited or occur spontaneously. They can be transmitted to following generations and cause disease in offspring. Some gene mutations can be silent (not causing a disease), some may skip generations, and some may affect males only. Mutation in the presenilin 1 gene is responsible for most of inherited, early-onset AD. This type of mutation almost always causes a disease if it is inherited.

Geriatrician: Internist specializing in medical problems of elderly individuals

Global deterioration scale: Scale used by physician to measure progression of AD

Glutamate: Activating neurotramitter abundant in the hippocampus and indispensable in the process of learning and making new memories

Gray matter: Part of the brain containing nerve cells. Brain cortex and basal ganglia are examples of gray matter. The term "gray matter" is derived from the natural color of this part of the brain.

Hallucinations: False notions of nonexisting objects or happenings. They may affect all senses; therefore, types include visual hallucination (seeing nonexisting things), sensory hallucination (feeling touch when nothing is touching), or auditory hallucination (hearing nonexisting voices). Hallucinations may also involve the senses of smell and taste.

Hamilton depression scale: Clinical scale used to measure severity of depression.

Hippocampus: Part of the brain responsible for learning and making new memories. In AD, it is the earliest structure to be most severely damaged, causing the obvious memory loss for which this disease is known.

Homocysteine: Product of normal body metabolism actively removed from the body. An elevated level of homocysteine is toxic.

Homocysteinemia: Increased level of homocysteine associated with increased risk for stroke, heart attack, and AD.

Huntington's disease: Inherited neurodegenerative disease associated with difficulty in controlling "dance-like" movements and eventually with dementia.

Hypercholesterolemia: Elevated level of cholesterol due to increased cholesterol intake, inherited predisposition, or both. Hypercholesterolemia is a risk factor for heart attack, stroke, and AD.

Hypertension: Elevated blood pressure occurring in every fourth person after age 50 and forming a significant risk factor for stroke and heart attack if untreated.

Hypothyroidism: Abnormally low function of the thyroid gland associated with slow metabolism, lower heart rate, cold intolerance, leg edema, and (in older people) symptoms of dementia.

Isoform: An alternate form of the same protein showing minute differences in chemical composition. For example, apoliprotein E may exist in three isoforms—E2, E3, and E4—in humans.

Lacunar infarction: Small brain infarction or stroke (less than 10 mm).

Lewy-body dementia: Form of dementia caused by degeneration of nerve cells that accumulate structures called Lewy bodies made up of α-synuclein.

Magnetic resonance imaging: Method of taking pictures of living brains that is used by doctors to diagnose and follow up brain disease and is based on the use of a high-power magnetic field

Meninges: Membranes surrounding and cushioning the brain

Meningitis: Inflammation of the membranes surrounding and protecting the brain; can be bacterial (caused by bacteria) or fungal (caused by fungus).

Metabolism: All chemical reactions taking place in a living organism.

Metabolite: Product of a chemical reaction taking place in the body.

Methylmalonic acid: Molecule associated with metabolism of vitamin B12. Measurement of its level is a more sensitive marker of vitamin B12 deficiency, the level of vitamin B12 itself.

Movement disorder: Disease in which the ability to perform normal movements is affected, although a patient's strength is normal. Movements can be too slow (as in Parkinson's disease) or too fast (as in Huntington's disease). The patient may have difficulties in performing complex movements, or movements can be affected by tremor.

Multifactorial disease: Disease with a likelihood of occurrence increased by numerous factors. Most sporadic diseases (e.g., sporadic AD) are multifactorial diseases. Severe head injuries, apoliprotein E4, and elevated cholesterol are examples of factors increasing odds for AD.

Multiinfarct dementia: Dementia resulting from numerous and repetitive strokes.

Mutation: Genetic defect that usually causes genetic disease and can happen spontaneously or be inherited from one parent.

Myocardial infarction: Damage or death of heart muscle due to restricted blood flow to that muscle (also called heart attack).

Nerve cells: Cells comprising the brain and connected by long processes that make communication between them possible.

Nerve cell processes: Connectors between nerve cells.

Neurodegenerative disease: Nerve cell–damaging disease associated with deposits of toxic proteins inside and outside nerve cells and leading to their death and dementia .

Neurofibrillary tangles: Abnormal structures formed inside nerve cells in AD. Their presence cause dysfunction of nerve cells and eventually kills them. Neurofibrillary tangles are composed of tau protein.

Neuroleptics: Class of medications used to treat hallucinations, delusions, and agitation in AD patients

Neuron: *See* nerve cells.

Neuropsychological testing: Series of tests measuring various intellectual functions (e.g., memory, language, intelligence, judgment, problem solving, spatial orientation, and others) and used in AD to detect and measure deficits in various areas of cognition and memory in particular.

Neurotransmitter: Chemical compound secreted at connections between nerve cells, either stimulatory or inhibitory neurotrasmitters. By producing the former, a nerve cell may stimulate another nerve cell, whereas by producing the latter, a nerve cell may brake activity of another nerve cell.

Neurotrophic growth factors: Substances that can stimulate nerve cells to grow their processes over long distances and form new connections with other nerve cells. Neurotrophic growth factors are indispensable for development of the brain. The possibility of their application in AD to restore damaged brain cells is currently under study.

Normal-pressure hydrocephalus: Disease associated with excess of cerebrospinal fluid and seen in progressing problems with walking, urinary continence, and eventually dementia. Normal-pressure hydrocephalus is treated by surgically placing a shunt designed to drain excess cerebrospinal fluid from the brain.

Osteoporosis: Weakening of bones usually associated with aging and brought on by hormonal changes taking place during menopause in women.

Otitis: Ear inflammation.

Otolaryngologist: Doctor specializing in treating ear, nose, and throat diseases.

Pace maker: Device implanted in certain patients with heart problems for controlling heart rate. Installing a pace maker prohibits the use of magnetic resonance imaging.

Parkinson's disease: Neurodegenerative disease striking mainly the motor system and leading to appearance of disabling tremor, stiffness, and difficulties in walking.

Pathogenic gene mutation: An abnormality in a gene (a fragment of DNA coding for a specific protein) resulting in the appearance of disease.

Phenylalanine: Amino acid that is a natural element found in many food products. Because it tastes sweet but has no calories, it is often used as a sugar substitute.

Plaques: Local buildup of amyloid-β in the brain of AD patients, damaging nerve cells and destroying connections between them.

Power of attorney: Legal term for a document in which a patient gives a trusted person legal authority to act on his or her behalf; usually given to manage assets or health-related issues or both.

Presbyacousis: Age-related hearing loss, especially to higher-frequency sounds (e.g., a kettle whistle), that is extremely common in the elderly and helped by use of a hearing aid.

Presenilin 1 (PS1) and Presenilin 2 (PS2): Proteins associated with function of γ-secretase (amyloid-β-releasing enzyme). Their inherited defects (mutations) are responsible for the majority of familial cases of AD (the form of AD affecting many members of the same family before age of 65).

Primary progressive aphasia: Rare form of neurodegenerative disease leading to dementia in which the primary and leading problem is associated with language dysfunction. Patients with primary progressive aphasia slowly but steadily lose their ability to understand language and the meaning of particular words and ability to speak. They eventually become mute.

Progressive supranuclear palsy: Rare form of neurodegenerative disease resembling Parkinson's disease but, unlike Parkinson's disease, producing problems with directing gaze downward, frequent falls, and eventual severe problems with swallowing.

Psychotherapy: Therapy based on a conversations between patient and therapist (frequently a psychiatrist) to understand the mechanism of psychological distress related to a mental illness (e.g., depression) and to create psychological countermeasures to combat it.

Pulmonary embolism: Serious medical condition caused by closing off a lung artery by an embolus. Symptoms include chest pain and breathing difficulties.

Radioisotope: Compound emitting radioactivity, therefore detectable by special camera. Radioisotopes are used for certain medical investigations (e.g., cysternogram) in evaluating normal-pressure hydrocephalus.

Saturated fatty acids: Elements abundant in red meat (e.g., pork or beef). Increased intake of saturated fatty acids is associated with elevated risk of atherosclerosis and, as a consequence, occurrence of stroke or heart attack. In contrast, unsaturated fatty acids are abundant in fish, and their consumption lowers risk of atherosclerosis.

Secretases-β and -γ: Enzymes responsible for cutting out amyloid-β from the amyloid precursor protein

Secretase inhibitors: Line of experimental drugs for AD currently under development and designed to inhibit function of β- or γ-secretases and thereby decrease the amount of amyloid-β produced.

Serotonin: Neurotransmitter that when lacking is associated with symptoms of depression (e.g., low mood, excessive feeling of guilt, slowness, changes in sleep and eating habits).

Serotonin reuptake inhibitors: Class of medication used to treat depression by increasing levels of serotonin

Shunt: Drainage device placed in the brain to remove excess cerebrospinal fluid and used to treat (among other disorders) normal-pressure hydrocephalus.

Sporadic disease: Disease not caused by a specific inherited genetic defect but possibly affecting every person with a greater or lesser chance.

Statins: Drugs lowering cholesterol level and thereby reducing risk of heart attack and stroke. Clinical studies designed to determine whether they may also slow the course of AD are ongoing.

Stem cells: Cells in the bone marrow that have the capacity of turning into other cells of the body.

Substantia nigra: Part of the brain severely affected in Parkinson's disease, causing tremor, slow movements, and disability in walking.

Susceptibility: Being sensitive to damage or disease.

Tau protein: Abnormal protein that in AD piles up inside nerve cells, forming neurofibrillary tangles that directly lead to death of nerve cells.

Testosterone: Male sexual hormone.

Thyroid hormones: Hormones secreted by thyroid gland and essential for maintaining proper metabolism of the body. Their deficiency may cause symptoms of dementia (among other symptoms) in the elderly.

Transgenic: Genetically altered.

Vascular dementia: Second type of dementia (after AD) caused either by numerous strokes or a slowly ongoing process of closing off small brain vessels.

White matter: Part of the brain containing processes of nerve cells (brain wiring). It is white as opposed to gray matter, which contains actual nerve cell bodies.

Index

Index